HIGH PROTEIN HIGH FIBER
MEAL PREP COOKBOOK

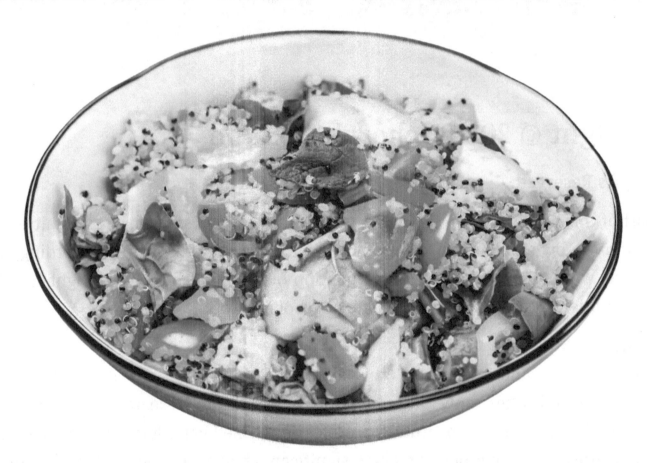

WHOLESOME RECIPES TO HELP YOU STAY NOURISHED, SATISFIED, AND ENERGIZED
THROUGHOUT THE DAY

DEBORAH DONOHO

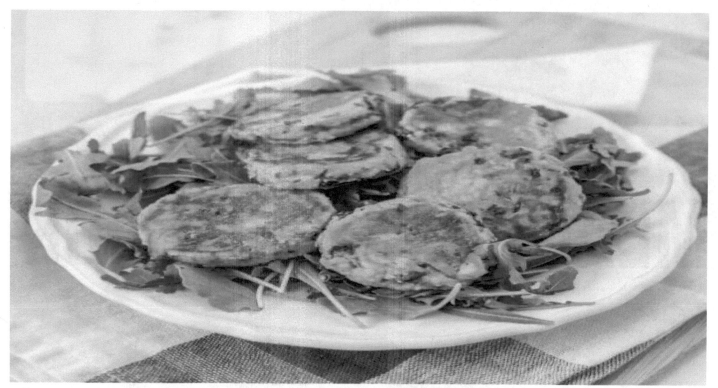

Copyright © 2025 Deborah Donoho

Disclaimer:

The information and recipes in this book are intended for educational and informational purposes only. The content is based on research and personal experience but does not substitute for professional medical advice. Always consult with a healthcare provider before making significant changes to your diet, especially if you have specific health conditions or concerns.

The author and publisher do not assume any responsibility for errors or omissions, or any adverse effects resulting from the use or application of any information or recipes contained in this book. The recipes are provided with the understanding that the author is not rendering medical, nutritional, or dietary advice.

TABLE OF CONTENTS

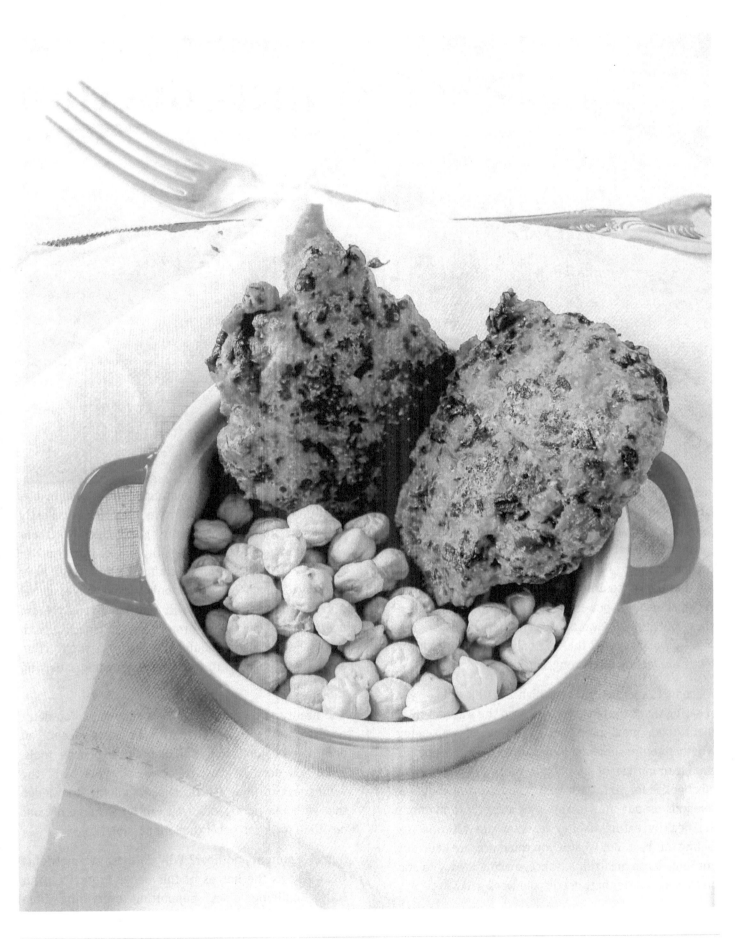

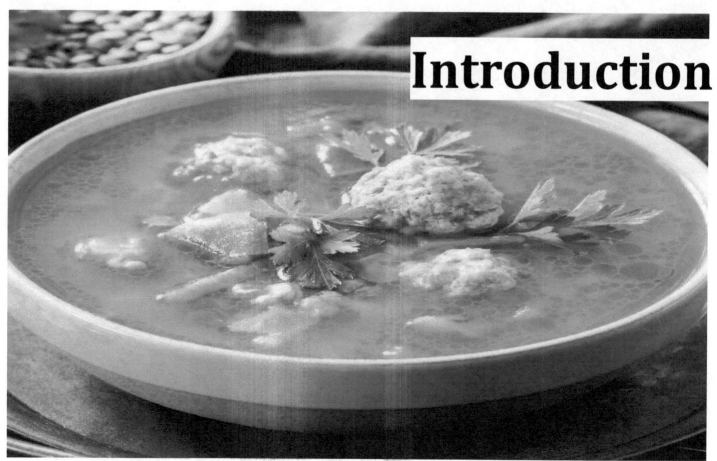

Introduction

Imagine waking up every day feeling energized, satisfied, and ready to take on whatever challenges come your way. No more midday slumps, no more endless cravings for snacks, and no more spending hours in the kitchen trying to figure out what to eat. What if I told you that the key to unlocking this version of yourself lies in two simple, yet powerful nutrients: protein and fiber? These nutritional powerhouses are the foundation for a healthy, balanced diet that not only fuels your body but keeps you feeling full, strong, and vibrant.

Welcome to the high-protein, high-fiber lifestyle—a way of eating that's designed to transform the way you think about food, meal prep, and your overall well-being. Whether you're someone looking to shed a few pounds, build lean muscle, or simply take control of your health, this book is for you. With busy schedules and countless demands on our time, many of us struggle to maintain the healthy eating habits we know are essential for feeling our best. But what if you could prepare delicious, nutrient-dense meals in advance, making it easy to stay on track no matter how hectic your week gets?

This cookbook is your ultimate guide to a sustainable, high-protein, high-fiber lifestyle that fits seamlessly into your routine. No more guesswork. No more resorting to fast food or unhealthy snacks when hunger strikes. With these carefully crafted recipes, you'll have an array of meals that are not only packed with essential nutrients but also bursting with flavor and variety. From hearty grain bowls to protein-packed snacks, from savory stews to indulgent desserts—you'll find everything you need to fuel your body while satisfying your taste buds.

The beauty of this approach is its simplicity. You don't need to be a gourmet chef to make these meals. You don't need complicated ingredients or expensive tools. What you need is a desire to nourish your body, the willingness to plan a little ahead, and the knowledge that with the right foods, you can take charge of your health in ways you never thought possible.

But why protein and fiber? Why do these two nutrients stand out as the heroes of this book? Protein is your body's building block, supporting everything from muscle repair to hormone regulation. It keeps you full, helps stabilize blood sugar levels, and plays a vital role in metabolism. Fiber, on the other hand, is your digestive system's best friend. It aids in digestion, promotes gut health, and keeps you feeling full and satisfied for longer periods of time—key to avoiding those pesky energy crashes and cravings.

Yet, despite their importance, many people struggle to get enough of these essential nutrients in their daily diets. That's where meal prep comes in. By planning ahead and prepping your meals, you can ensure that each day is packed with protein-rich, fiber-filled dishes that taste amazing and make healthy eating feel effortless.

In this book, you'll find more than just recipes. You'll discover how meal prepping can simplify your life, reduce food waste, and help you save money, all while supporting your nutritional goals. You'll learn how to create meals that are balanced, satisfying, and easy to adjust based on your personal preferences and dietary needs. From plant-based proteins to hearty legumes, from fresh vegetables to whole grains, this book will show you how to create meals that nourish your body, fuel your lifestyle, and fit seamlessly into your routine.

So whether you're new to meal prep or a seasoned pro looking for fresh ideas, this book is here to inspire you. It's time to take control of your health, simplify your life, and discover just how easy it can be to enjoy a high-protein, high-fiber lifestyle that helps you feel your best every single day.

Let's get started on the path to better nutrition, easier meal prep, and a healthier, happier you!

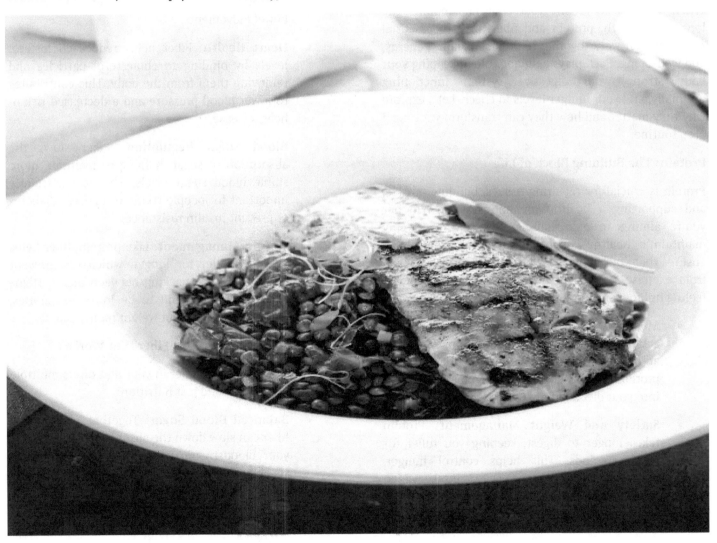

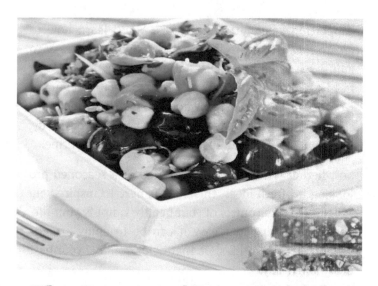

The Power of Protein and Fiber: Why They Matter

When it comes to fueling your body and maintaining long-term health, protein and fiber are two essential nutrients that work together to provide balance, energy, and well-being. Each plays a unique role in keeping your body strong, your digestive system functioning optimally, and your hunger levels in check. Let's explore why they matter and how they can transform your meal prep routine.

Protein: The Building Block of Life

Protein is crucial for repairing tissues, building muscle, and supporting a healthy immune system. Whether you're aiming to gain muscle, lose fat, or simply maintain a healthy weight, adequate protein intake ensures that your body has the tools it needs to recover from exercise, build lean muscle mass, and keep you feeling full longer. Here's why it's important:

- **Muscle Repair and Growth**: After physical activity, your muscles need protein to rebuild and grow stronger. Incorporating high-quality proteins like chicken, fish, legumes, and tofu into your diet supports this process.

- **Satiety and Weight Management**: Protein takes longer to digest, keeping you fuller for longer periods. This helps control hunger, making it easier to manage calorie intake, which is key for weight loss and maintaining a healthy weight.

- **Metabolism Boost**: Protein has a higher thermic effect of food (TEF) compared to fats and carbohydrates. This means your body uses more energy to digest and metabolize protein, effectively boosting your metabolism.

Fiber: The Unsung Hero of Digestion

Fiber plays an equally important role, especially when it comes to digestion and overall gut health. It's the part of plant-based foods that your body can't digest, but it's vital for moving food through the digestive system and maintaining blood sugar levels. Here's why fiber is essential:

- **Improved Digestion**: Soluble fiber helps to slow down digestion, allowing your body to absorb more nutrients from the food you eat. Insoluble fiber adds bulk to your stool, helping prevent constipation and promoting regular bowel movements.

- **Heart Health**: Fiber helps reduce cholesterol levels by binding to cholesterol particles and removing them from the body. This contributes to lower blood pressure and a decreased risk of heart disease.

- **Blood Sugar Regulation**: Fiber slows the absorption of sugar, helping to maintain more stable blood sugar levels. This is particularly important for people trying to manage diabetes or prevent insulin resistance.

- **Weight Management**: Like protein, fiber helps you feel fuller for longer, which can prevent overeating and snacking between meals. High-fiber foods also tend to be lower in calories, making them great for weight management.

Why a High-Protein, High-Fiber Diet Works

Combining protein and fiber in your diet offers multiple benefits that go beyond just nutrition:

- **Balanced Blood Sugar**: Together, protein and fiber can slow down the absorption of sugar into your bloodstream, which helps prevent blood sugar spikes and crashes, keeping your energy levels stable.

- **Sustained Fullness**: Both protein and fiber promote satiety, meaning you'll feel fuller for longer. This can help reduce overall calorie intake and make it easier to stick to healthy eating habits.

- **Nutrient Density**: A high-protein, high-fiber diet typically involves nutrient-dense foods like lean meats, legumes, whole grains, and vegetables, which provide a wide range of vitamins and minerals essential for overall health.

The Next Step: Putting It Into Practice

Understanding the power of protein and fiber is one thing but applying it to your meal prep is the real game-changer. By incorporating high-protein, high-fiber meals into your weekly routine, you'll find that you have more energy, stay full longer, and can reach your fitness and wellness goals with more ease.

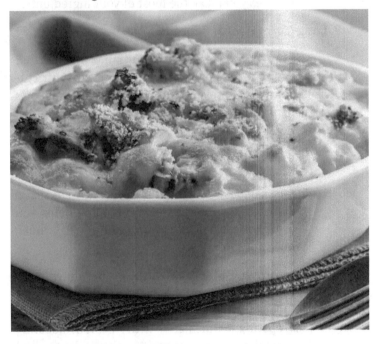

How Meal Prep Transforms Your Health

Meal prepping is more than just a time-saver; it's a powerful strategy that can significantly impact your overall health and well-being. By planning and preparing your meals ahead of time, you're not only setting yourself up for success in the kitchen but also creating a foundation for healthier habits, better nutrition, and long-term lifestyle changes.

Here's how meal prepping can transform your health:

1. Better Portion Control and Calorie Management

One of the biggest advantages of meal prep is the ability to control portions and monitor your calorie intake with precision. When meals are planned in advance, you're less likely to indulge in oversized portions or eat impulsively. This is especially beneficial for those aiming for weight loss, muscle gain, or maintaining a healthy weight.

- **Pre-measured Portions**: By dividing meals into appropriate portions, you ensure that every meal is balanced and aligned with your health goals. This eliminates the guesswork and keeps your nutrition on track.

- **Calorie Awareness**: Prepping meals gives you full control over the ingredients and cooking methods, allowing you to easily adjust calories and macronutrient ratios based on your goals.

2. Consistency and Commitment to Healthy Eating

Meal prepping helps you stay consistent with your dietary habits, which is crucial for achieving long-term health goals. When healthy meals are ready to go, you're less likely to make poor food choices or reach for convenient, processed options.

- **Avoiding Temptation**: When you're hungry and unprepared, it's easy to grab fast food or snack on unhealthy options. Meal prep ensures that you always have nutritious meals within reach, minimizing the likelihood of impulsive eating.

- **Creating Healthy Habits**: The routine of meal prepping promotes discipline and makes it easier to stick to your dietary plan. Over time, this consistency translates into lasting lifestyle changes.

3. Improved Nutritional Quality

When you cook your own meals, you have complete control over the ingredients, allowing you to choose healthier, nutrient-dense foods that support your well-being. Meal prepping encourages you to focus on whole foods like lean proteins, whole grains, vegetables, and healthy fats, which naturally improve the quality of your diet.

- **Avoiding Processed Foods**: Prepping meals at home helps you avoid processed and packaged foods, which are often high in sodium, unhealthy fats, and preservatives.

- **Balanced Nutrition**: When you plan your meals in advance, it's easier to ensure that each meal contains a balanced mix of protein, fiber, healthy fats, and essential vitamins and minerals.

4. Reducing Stress and Anxiety Around Food

Making daily food choices can be stressful, especially when you're trying to eat healthy in a busy, fast-paced life. Meal prepping takes the guesswork out of what to eat, reducing decision fatigue and the anxiety that often comes with last-minute meal planning.

- **Planning Ahead = Less Stress**: When your meals are already prepared, you can avoid the daily stress of figuring out what to eat. This frees up mental energy for other important areas of your life.

- **Confidence in Your Diet**: Knowing that you have nutritious meals planned gives you peace of mind and confidence that you're nourishing your body well, which can reduce the guilt or stress associated with unhealthy eating.

5. Supporting Fitness and Weight Goals

Whether your goal is to build muscle, lose weight, or improve your overall fitness, meal prep plays a crucial role in supporting those efforts. By carefully planning your meals, you can ensure that you're eating the right nutrients in the right quantities to fuel your workouts and recovery.

- **Customized to Your Goals**: Meal prepping allows you to tailor your meals to specific fitness objectives—whether that's increasing protein intake for muscle gain or managing calories for fat loss.

- **Recovery and Energy**: Preparing balanced meals in advance ensures that you have the right nutrients to recover after workouts, stay energized throughout the day, and prevent overeating.

6. Saving Time and Money

Meal prepping not only improves your health but also saves you time and money in the long run. By cooking in bulk and planning your grocery list, you avoid unnecessary purchases and reduce food waste, making meal prep both cost-effective and efficient.

- **Batch Cooking**: Preparing meals in larger quantities means fewer cooking sessions and more free time during the week. Plus, having pre-cooked meals in the fridge or freezer cuts down on the temptation to order takeout, saving you money.

- **Grocery Efficiency**: Meal prepping encourages you to stick to a grocery list, buying only what you need. This minimizes impulse buys and ensures you make the most of your ingredients.

7. Long-Term Health Benefits

By meal prepping regularly, you build habits that promote long-term health. A well-balanced, nutrient-dense diet helps prevent chronic diseases, supports mental health, and contributes to an overall sense of well-being.

- **Preventing Chronic Diseases**: Diets high in processed foods, refined sugars, and unhealthy fats can lead to conditions like heart disease, diabetes, and obesity. Meal prepping helps you avoid these risks by focusing on whole, nutritious foods.

- **Improving Mental Health**: Proper nutrition is linked to better mood, mental clarity, and reduced symptoms of anxiety and depression. Preparing meals with brain-boosting ingredients like omega-3s, antioxidants, and fiber can support your mental health.

Getting Started with Meal Prepping: Planning Ahead for Success

Meal prepping is a game-changer when it comes to maintaining a healthy diet and saving time during the week. But if you're new to meal prepping, it can feel a little overwhelming at first. The key to success is planning ahead and breaking the process down into manageable steps. Here's how to get started:

1. Set Clear Goals

Before diving into meal prepping, it's important to clarify your health goals. Whether you're aiming to lose weight, build muscle, improve overall nutrition, or simply save time, having a clear objective will guide your planning and recipe choices.

- **Health and Fitness Goals**: Do you need meals that support muscle growth, weight loss, or a specific dietary requirement (e.g., high-protein, low-carb)?

- **Time Management**: Are you prepping meals for the entire week, or just a few days? Decide how much time you want to dedicate to meal prepping.

Once you know your goals, you can tailor your meal prep strategy to meet them, ensuring you're focusing on the right balance of nutrients and portion sizes.

2. Plan Your Weekly Menu

The most efficient meal preppers always start with a plan. Before heading to the grocery store or cooking, map out what you're going to eat for the week. This saves time, reduces food waste, and ensures you're eating a balanced diet.

- **Choose Recipes**: Pick meals that fit your dietary goals, are easy to prep in bulk, and reheat well. Variety is key to avoiding meal fatigue, so try to mix things up with different flavors and cuisines.

- **Balance Macronutrients**: Make sure your weekly menu includes a good balance of proteins, fiber-rich carbs, and healthy fats. You can reference the previous section on building balanced meals to help guide your choices.

- **Include Snacks**: Don't forget to plan for high-protein, high-fiber snacks. Having healthy options on hand can help curb cravings and prevent you from reaching for unhealthy foods.

3. Make a Detailed Shopping List

Once your menu is set, create a shopping list that includes everything you need for your meal prep. This ensures you have all the ingredients on hand when you start cooking and prevents impulse purchases that could derail your healthy eating plan.

- **Organize by Category**: Divide your shopping list into categories like proteins, vegetables, grains, and pantry staples to make your trip to the store more efficient.

- **Stick to Your List**: Avoid buying extra items that aren't part of your plan. Sticking to your list helps you stay within budget and reduces the temptation to purchase unhealthy foods.

4. Set Aside Time for Meal Prep

Successful meal prepping requires setting aside dedicated time. Most people choose to prep on weekends, but the best time is whenever you can carve out a couple of hours for cooking.

- **Batch Cooking**: Cooking in larger quantities saves time and ensures you have enough food for the week. For example, you can roast a big tray of vegetables or cook a large batch of grains to use in multiple meals.

- **Multitask**: While something is baking in the oven, you can be chopping vegetables, cooking grains, or preparing proteins on the stovetop. Maximize your time by working on multiple components at once.

5. Invest in the Right Storage Solutions

Having the right containers can make a huge difference in how easy meal prep is, and it also helps keep your meals fresh throughout the week.

- **Meal Prep Containers**: Invest in high-quality, BPA-free plastic or glass containers that are microwave and dishwasher-safe. Choose containers with compartments for separating different meal components (e.g., proteins and vegetables).

- **Label and Date**: Label your containers with the meal and the date it was prepped. This helps you stay organized and ensures you eat meals while they're still fresh.

6. Start Small and Build Momentum

If you're new to meal prepping, it's important to start small. You don't need to prep all your meals for the week at once. Instead, focus on one or two meals to begin with—like prepping lunches or dinners in advance.

- **Choose Easy, Flexible Recipes**: Start with simple recipes that don't require too many ingredients or steps. Once you're comfortable, you can expand your repertoire and begin prepping for more meals.

- **Adjust as You Go**: Your first week may not be perfect, and that's okay. Keep adjusting your meal prep routine based on what works for you—whether it's adjusting portion sizes, prep time, or the types of meals you're making.

7. Keep Your Pantry and Freezer Stocked

One of the best ways to make meal prepping easier is to keep your pantry and freezer stocked with healthy staples that you can rely on when time is tight.

- **Pantry Staples**: Stock up on grains like quinoa, brown rice, oats, and legumes. Keep a variety of spices, canned goods (like beans and tomatoes), and healthy oils on hand.

- **Freezer Staples**: Frozen vegetables, pre-cooked proteins (like grilled chicken or tofu), and cooked grains can be life-savers when you need to throw together a meal quickly. You can also freeze pre-prepped meals for busy weeks when you won't have time to cook.

8. Monitor and Adjust

Meal prepping is a process, and it may take a few tries before you find your rhythm. Pay attention to how much food you're eating, how well your meals reheat, and whether you're enjoying the meals you've prepped. Adjust recipes, portion sizes, and prep frequency as needed.

- **Listen to Your Body**: If a certain meal doesn't keep you full or energized, make a note and adjust the protein, fiber, or fat content for next time.

- **Don't Be Afraid to Switch It Up**: Meal prep should be enjoyable and sustainable, so keep experimenting with new flavors, ingredients, and recipes to keep things interesting.

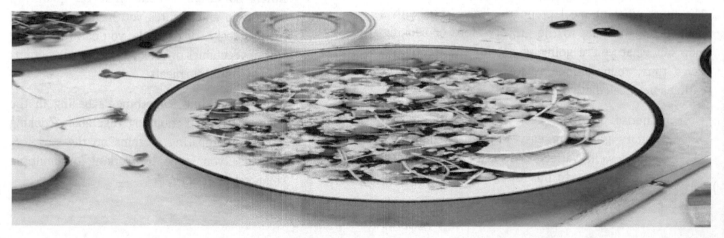

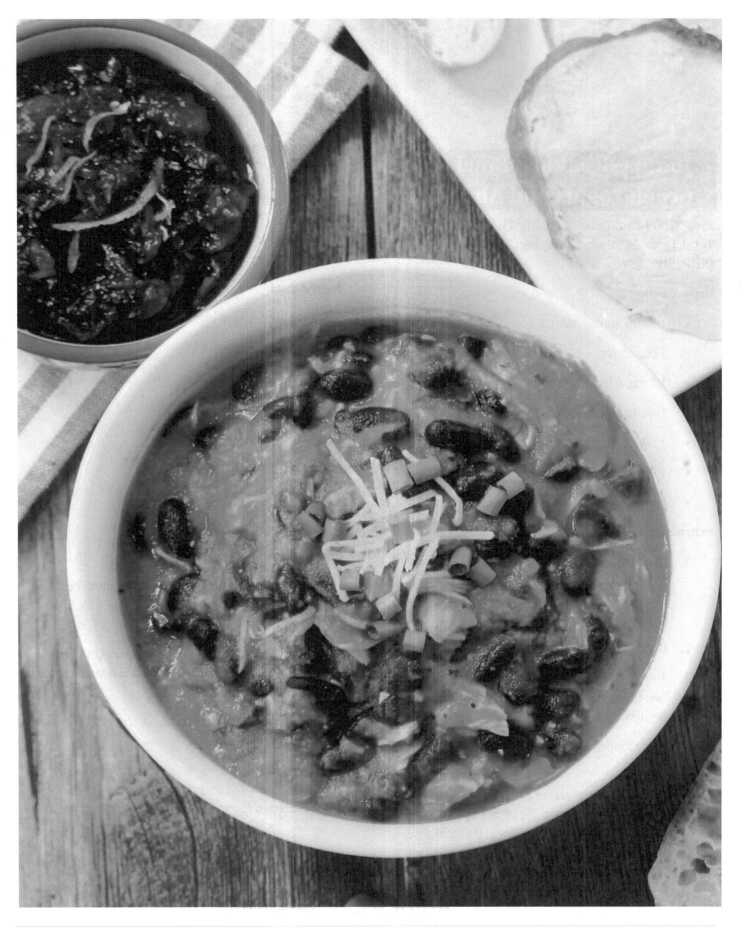

Breakfast

Quinoa Breakfast Bowl with Greek Yogurt and Almonds

Prep Time: 10 minutes | **Cooking Time:** 15 minutes | **Total Time:** 25 minutes | **Serving:** 2 | **Cooking Difficulty:** Easy

Ingredients:

- 1/2 cup quinoa, rinsed
- 1 cup water
- 1/2 cup Greek yogurt
- 1/4 cup almonds, sliced
- 1 tablespoon honey or maple syrup
- 1/2 teaspoon cinnamon
- Fresh berries (optional, for topping)

Instructions:

1. In a medium saucepan, bring quinoa and water to a boil. Reduce heat, cover, and simmer for about 12-15 minutes until water is absorbed and quinoa is cooked. Fluff with a fork.
2. Divide quinoa into two bowls.
3. Top each bowl with Greek yogurt, almonds, honey, and cinnamon. Add fresh berries if desired.
4. Serve immediately.

Nutritional Value:

Calories 250 | Fat 7g | Saturated Fat 1g | Cholesterol 5mg | Sodium 25mg | Carbohydrate 38g | Fiber 5g | Added Sugar 6g | Protein 12g | Calcium 120mg | Potassium 300mg | Iron 1.8mg | Vitamin D 0mcg

Black Bean and Egg White Burrito

Prep Time: 10 minutes | **Cooking Time:** 10 minutes | **Total Time:** 20 minutes | **Serving:** 4 | **Cooking Difficulty:** Easy

Ingredients:

- 1 cup canned black beans, drained and rinsed
- 4 large egg whites
- 1/4 cup diced bell peppers
- 1/4 cup diced onions
- 1/2 teaspoon cumin
- 1/2 teaspoon paprika
- 4 whole-wheat tortillas
- Salsa, for serving (optional)

Instructions:

1. Heat a non-stick skillet over medium heat and add bell peppers and onions. Sauté for 3-4 minutes until soft.
2. Add black beans, cumin, and paprika to the skillet. Stir until combined and heated through, about 2 minutes.
3. In a separate pan, scramble the egg whites until fully cooked.
4. Assemble the burritos by placing the bean mixture and scrambled egg whites in the center of each tortilla. Fold and roll into burritos.
5. Serve with salsa on the side, if desired.

Nutritional Value:

Calories 200 | Fat 4g | Saturated Fat 0.5g | Cholesterol

0mg | Sodium 320mg | Carbohydrate 30g | Fiber 7g | Added Sugar 1g | Protein 12g | Calcium 70mg | Potassium 400mg | Iron 2.5mg | Vitamin D 0mcg

Chickpea Flour Pancakes

Prep Time: 5 minutes | **Cooking Time**: 15 minutes | **Total Time**: 20 minutes | **Serving**: 2 | **Cooking Difficulty**: Moderate

Ingredients:

- 1 cup chickpea flour
- 1/2 cup water
- 1/4 teaspoon turmeric powder
- 1/4 teaspoon cumin powder
- 1/4 teaspoon salt
- 1/2 cup chopped spinach
- 1/4 cup grated carrots
- 1 tablespoon olive oil (for cooking)

Instructions:

1. In a mixing bowl, whisk together chickpea flour, water, turmeric, cumin, and salt until a smooth batter forms.
2. Stir in chopped spinach and grated carrots.
3. Heat a non-stick pan over medium heat and add a little olive oil.
4. Pour about 1/4 cup of batter onto the pan, forming a pancake. Cook for 3-4 minutes on each side until golden brown and cooked through.
5. Repeat with remaining batter. Serve warm.

Nutritional Value:
Calories 210 | Fat 7g | Saturated Fat 1g | Cholesterol 0mg | Sodium 380mg | Carbohydrate 29g | Fiber 5g | Added Sugar 0g | Protein 9g | Calcium 50mg | Potassium 350mg | Iron 2.5mg | Vitamin D 0mcg

Lentil and Spinach Breakfast Patties

Prep Time: 10 minutes | **Cooking Time**: 20 minutes | **Total Time**: 30 minutes | **Serving**: 4 | **Cooking Difficulty**: Moderate

Ingredients:

- 1 cup cooked lentils
- 1/2 cup finely chopped spinach
- 1/4 cup breadcrumbs (whole wheat or gluten-free)
- 1 egg (or flax egg for vegan)
- 1/2 teaspoon garlic powder
- 1/2 teaspoon onion powder
- 1/4 teaspoon cumin
- 1 tablespoon olive oil (for frying)

Instructions:

1. In a large bowl, combine cooked lentils, spinach, breadcrumbs, egg, garlic powder, onion powder, and cumin.
2. Form the mixture into small patties (about 8).
3. Heat olive oil in a skillet over medium heat and cook the patties for about 3-4 minutes on each side until golden brown and heated through.
4. Serve warm, with a side of yogurt or salsa.

Nutritional Value:
Calories 180 | Fat 6g | Saturated Fat 1g | Cholesterol 35mg | Sodium 220mg | Carbohydrate 23g | Fiber 6g | Added Sugar 0g | Protein 8g | Calcium 50mg | Potassium 300mg | Iron 2mg | Vitamin D 0mcg

Chia Seed Protein Pudding

Prep Time: 5 minutes (plus chilling time) | **Cooking Time**: 0 minutes | **Total Time**: 5 minutes (plus 4 hours chilling) | **Serving**: 2 | **Cooking Difficulty**: Easy

Ingredients:

- 1/4 cup chia seeds
- 1 cup almond milk (or any milk of choice)
- 1 scoop vanilla protein powder
- 1 tablespoon maple syrup or honey (optional)
- Fresh berries, for topping

Instructions:

1. In a medium bowl, whisk together chia seeds, almond milk, protein powder, and maple syrup until well combined.

2. Let the mixture sit for 5 minutes, then stir again to prevent clumping.

3. Cover and refrigerate for at least 4 hours or overnight, until the mixture thickens to a pudding-like consistency.

4. Serve chilled, topped with fresh berries if desired.

Nutritional Value:
Calories 240 | Fat 8g | Saturated Fat 1g | Cholesterol 0mg | Sodium 150mg | Carbohydrate 28g | Fiber 10g | Added Sugar 6g | Protein 15g | Calcium 300mg | Potassium 350mg | Iron 2.1mg | Vitamin D 0mcg

Steel Cut Oats with Hemp Seeds and Berries

Prep Time: 5 minutes | **Cooking Time**: 25 minutes | **Total Time**: 30 minutes | **Serving**: 2 | **Cooking Difficulty**: Easy

Ingredients:

- 1/2 cup steel-cut oats
- 2 cups water
- 1 tablespoon hemp seeds
- 1/2 cup fresh mixed berries (blueberries, raspberries, strawberries)
- 1 tablespoon honey or maple syrup (optional)
- 1/4 teaspoon cinnamon
- 1/4 teaspoon vanilla extract (optional)

Instructions:

1. In a medium saucepan, bring water to a boil. Add the steel-cut oats, reduce heat to low, and simmer for 20-25 minutes, stirring occasionally, until the oats are tender and the water is absorbed.

2. Remove from heat and stir in cinnamon and vanilla extract if using.

3. Divide oats into bowls and top with hemp seeds, fresh berries, and a drizzle of honey or maple syrup, if desired.

4. Serve warm.

Nutritional Value:
Calories 240 | Fat 6g | Saturated Fat 1g | Cholesterol 0mg | Sodium 5mg | Carbohydrate 41g | Fiber 8g | Added Sugar 5g | Protein 8g | Calcium 50mg | Potassium 200mg | Iron 2.2mg | Vitamin D 0mcg

Tempeh Breakfast Scramble

Prep Time: 10 minutes | **Cooking Time:** 15 minutes | **Total Time:** 25 minutes | **Serving:** 2 | **Cooking Difficulty:** Moderate

Ingredients:

- 1 (8-ounce) block tempeh, crumbled
- 1/2 red bell pepper, diced
- 1/2 onion, diced
- 1/2 teaspoon turmeric powder
- 1/4 teaspoon cumin powder
- 1/4 teaspoon garlic powder
- 1 tablespoon olive oil
- Salt and pepper, to taste
- Fresh parsley, chopped (optional, for garnish)

Instructions:

1. Heat olive oil in a skillet over medium heat. Add diced onion and bell pepper, sauté for 4-5 minutes until softened.
2. Add crumbled tempeh to the skillet along with turmeric, cumin, garlic powder, salt, and pepper. Cook for 8-10 minutes, stirring occasionally, until the tempeh is heated through and slightly crispy.
3. Adjust seasoning to taste.
4. Garnish with chopped parsley and serve warm.

Nutritional Value:

Calories 260 | Fat 12g | Saturated Fat 2g | Cholesterol 0mg | Sodium 350mg | Carbohydrate 19g | Fiber 5g | Added Sugar 0g | Protein 21g | Calcium 80mg | Potassium 400mg | Iron 3mg | Vitamin D 0mcg

Black Bean Breakfast Bowl

Prep Time: 10 minutes | **Cooking Time:** 10 minutes | **Total Time:** 20 minutes | **Serving:** 2 | **Cooking Difficulty:** Easy

Ingredients:

- 1 can (15 ounces) black beans, drained and rinsed
- 1/2 cup cooked quinoa
- 1/2 avocado, sliced
- 1/4 cup salsa
- 2 tablespoons shredded cheddar cheese (optional)
- 1/4 teaspoon cumin
- 1/4 teaspoon paprika
- 1 tablespoon olive oil
- Salt and pepper, to taste

Instructions:

1. In a skillet, heat olive oil over medium heat. Add black beans, cumin, paprika, salt, and pepper, and cook for 3-4 minutes until beans are heated through.
2. Divide the cooked quinoa between two bowls.
3. Top each bowl with the black beans, avocado slices, salsa, and shredded cheddar cheese if using.
4. Serve warm.

Nutritional Value:

Calories 350 | Fat 16g | Saturated Fat 3g | Cholesterol 5mg | Sodium 400mg | Carbohydrate 42g | Fiber 12g | Added Sugar 0g | Protein 13g | Calcium 100mg | Potassium 600mg | Iron 3.5mg | Vitamin D 0mcg

Protein-Packed Overnight Oats

Prep Time: 5 minutes (plus chilling time) | **Cooking Time:** 0 minutes | **Total Time:** 5 minutes (plus overnight) | **Serving:** 2 | **Cooking Difficulty:** Easy

Ingredients:

- 1/2 cup rolled oats
- 1 scoop vanilla protein powder
- 1 tablespoon chia seeds
- 1/2 cup almond milk (or any milk of choice)
- 1/4 cup Greek yogurt
- 1/4 teaspoon cinnamon
- Fresh berries (optional, for topping)

Instructions:

1. In a mason jar or bowl, combine oats, protein powder, chia seeds, almond milk, Greek yogurt, and cinnamon.
2. Stir well to combine. Cover and refrigerate overnight or for at least 4 hours.
3. In the morning, stir again and top with fresh berries if desired.
4. Serve chilled.

Nutritional Value:
Calories 280 | Fat 7g | Saturated Fat 1g | Cholesterol 5mg | Sodium 140mg | Carbohydrate 36g | Fiber 8g | Added Sugar 3g | Protein 22g | Calcium 250mg | Potassium 300mg | Iron 2mg | Vitamin D 0mcg

Edamame Toast with Poached Eggs

Prep Time: 10 minutes | **Cooking Time:** 10 minutes | **Total Time:** 20 minutes | **Serving:** 2 | **Cooking Difficulty:** Moderate

Ingredients:

- 2 slices whole-grain bread, toasted
- 1/2 cup shelled edamame (cooked)
- 2 large eggs
- 1 tablespoon lemon juice
- 1 tablespoon olive oil
- Salt and pepper, to taste
- Fresh parsley, chopped (optional, for garnish)

Instructions:

1. In a food processor, pulse the cooked edamame with lemon juice, olive oil, salt, and pepper until smooth.
2. Spread the edamame mixture evenly on the toasted whole-grain bread slices.
3. Bring a small pot of water to a simmer and poach the eggs for 3-4 minutes until the whites are set but the yolks are still runny.
4. Top each toast with a poached egg, season with salt and pepper, and garnish with parsley if desired.
5. Serve immediately.

Nutritional Value:
Calories 300 | Fat 15g | Saturated Fat 3g | Cholesterol 185mg | Sodium 240mg | Carbohydrate 25g | Fiber 6g | Added Sugar 0g | Protein 18g | Calcium 80mg | Potassium 400mg | Iron 3mg | Vitamin D 1.2mcg

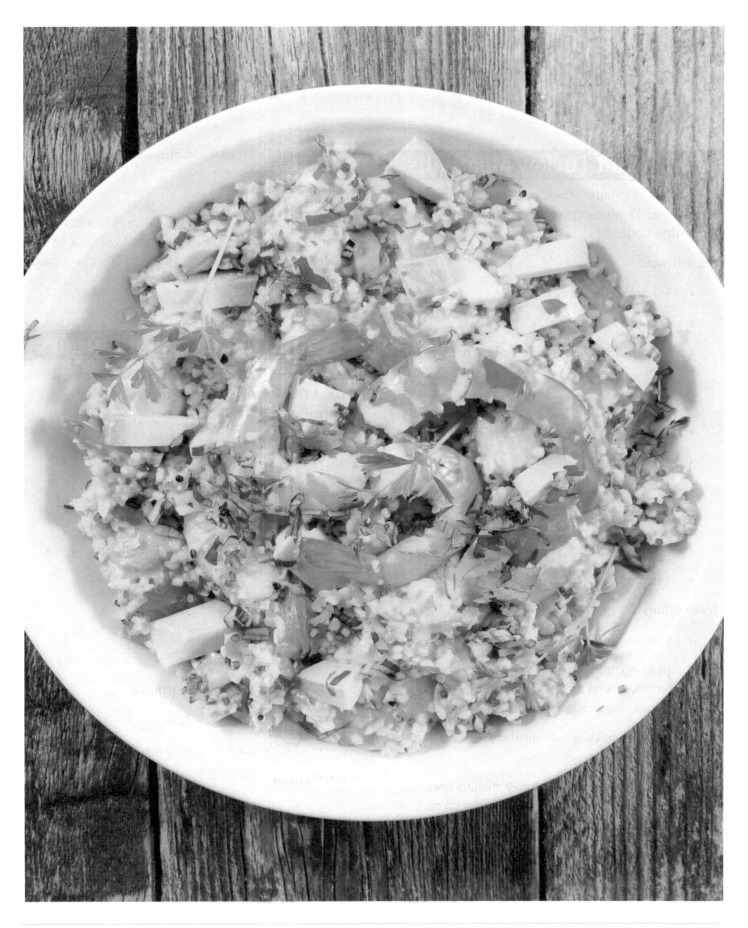

Main Dishes

Lentil and Turkey Meatballs

Prep Time: 15 minutes | **Cooking Time**: 20 minutes | **Total Time**: 35 minutes | **Serving**: 4 | **Cooking Difficulty**: Moderate

Ingredients:

- 1/2 cup cooked lentils
- 1/2 pound ground turkey
- 1/4 cup breadcrumbs (whole wheat or gluten-free)
- 1 egg
- 1 clove garlic, minced
- 1/4 teaspoon cumin
- 1/4 teaspoon oregano
- 1/4 teaspoon salt
- 1/4 teaspoon black pepper
- 1 tablespoon olive oil (for cooking)

Instructions:

1. Preheat the oven to 400°F (200°C).

2. In a large mixing bowl, combine the cooked lentils, ground turkey, breadcrumbs, egg, garlic, cumin, oregano, salt, and pepper. Mix well.

3. Form the mixture into small meatballs (about 16).

4. Heat olive oil in a skillet over medium heat. Brown the meatballs for 2-3 minutes on each side, then transfer them to a baking sheet.

5. Bake in the oven for 15-18 minutes until fully cooked through.

6. Serve with your favorite sauce or over a bed of vegetables.

Nutritional Value:

Calories 220 | Fat 9g | Saturated Fat 2g | Cholesterol 85mg | Sodium 320mg | Carbohydrate 15g | Fiber 4g | Added Sugar 0g | Protein 22g | Calcium 50mg | Potassium 350mg | Iron 2mg | Vitamin D 0.5mcg

Quinoa Black Bean Burgers

Prep Time: 15 minutes | **Cooking Time**: 15 minutes | **Total Time**: 30 minutes | **Serving**: 4 | **Cooking Difficulty**: Moderate

Ingredients:

- 1/2 cup cooked quinoa
- 1 can (15 ounces) black beans, drained and rinsed
- 1/4 cup breadcrumbs (whole wheat or gluten-free)
- 1/2 small onion, diced
- 1 clove garlic, minced
- 1/4 teaspoon cumin
- 1/4 teaspoon smoked paprika
- Salt and pepper, to taste
- 1 tablespoon olive oil (for cooking)

Instructions:

1. In a large mixing bowl, mash the black beans with a fork or potato masher until mostly smooth.

2. Add the cooked quinoa, breadcrumbs, diced onion, garlic, cumin, smoked paprika, salt, and pepper. Mix until well combined.

3. Form the mixture into 4 patties.

4. Heat olive oil in a skillet over medium heat. Cook the patties for 4-5 minutes on each side until golden brown and heated through.

5. Serve on whole-grain buns or lettuce wraps with your favorite toppings.

Nutritional Value:

Calories 290 | Fat 9g | Saturated Fat 1.5g | Cholesterol 0mg | Sodium 320mg | Carbohydrate 40g | Fiber 10g | Added Sugar 0g | Protein 12g | Calcium 60mg | Potassium 550mg | Iron 3.5mg | Vitamin D 0mcg

Chickpea and Chicken Curry

Prep Time: 10 minutes | **Cooking Time**: 25 minutes | **Total Time**: 35 minutes | **Serving**: 4 | **Cooking Difficulty**: Moderate

Ingredients:

- 1 pound boneless, skinless chicken breasts, diced

- 1 can (15 ounces) chickpeas, drained and rinsed

- 1 onion, chopped

- 1 tablespoon curry powder

- 1/2 teaspoon cumin

- 1/2 teaspoon turmeric

- 1 can (14 ounces) diced tomatoes

- 1 cup coconut milk (light or regular)

- 1 tablespoon olive oil

- Salt and pepper, to taste

- Fresh cilantro, for garnish (optional)

Instructions:

1. Heat olive oil in a large skillet over medium heat. Add the chopped onion and cook for 3-4 minutes until softened.

2. Add the diced chicken, curry powder, cumin, turmeric, salt, and pepper. Cook for 5-7 minutes until the chicken is browned.

3. Stir in the diced tomatoes, chickpeas, and coconut milk. Bring to a simmer and cook for 15 minutes until the sauce thickens and the chicken is fully cooked.

4. Garnish with fresh cilantro and serve over rice or quinoa.

Nutritional Value:

Calories 350 | Fat 14g | Saturated Fat 7g | Cholesterol 65mg | Sodium 420mg | Carbohydrate 28g | Fiber 6g | Added Sugar 0g | Protein 28g | Calcium 50mg | Potassium 700mg | Iron 3mg | Vitamin D 0mcg

Split Pea and Ham Soup

Prep Time: 10 minutes | **Cooking Time**: 1 hour | **Total Time**: 1 hour 10 minutes | **Serving**: 4 | **Cooking Difficulty**: Moderate

Ingredients:

- 1 cup dried split peas, rinsed

- 1 small onion, diced

- 1 carrot, diced

- 1 celery stalk, diced

- 1 cup diced ham

- 4 cups chicken broth (low sodium)

- 1/2 teaspoon thyme

- 1/4 teaspoon black pepper

- 1 tablespoon olive oil

- Salt, to taste

Instructions:

1. Heat olive oil in a large pot over medium heat. Add the onion, carrot, and celery, and cook for 5 minutes until softened.

2. Stir in the diced ham and cook for 2-3 minutes.

3. Add the split peas, chicken broth, thyme, and pepper. Bring to a boil, then reduce the heat and simmer for 1 hour, stirring occasionally, until the peas are tender and the soup thickens.

4. Season with salt to taste. Serve hot.

Nutritional Value:
Calories 280 | Fat 9g | Saturated Fat 2g | Cholesterol 40mg | Sodium 540mg | Carbohydrate 34g | Fiber 12g | Added Sugar 0g | Protein 19g | Calcium 40mg | Potassium 500mg | Iron 2mg | Vitamin D 0mcg

Three-Bean Turkey Chili

Prep Time: 10 minutes | **Cooking Time**: 30 minutes | **Total Time**: 40 minutes | **Serving**: 4 | **Cooking Difficulty**: Easy

Ingredients:

- 1 pound ground turkey

- 1 can (15 ounces) black beans, drained and rinsed

- 1 can (15 ounces) kidney beans, drained and rinsed

- 1 can (15 ounces) pinto beans, drained and rinsed

- 1 can (14 ounces) diced tomatoes

- 1 onion, diced

- 2 cloves garlic, minced

- 2 tablespoons chili powder

- 1 teaspoon cumin

- 1 teaspoon smoked paprika

- 1 tablespoon olive oil

- Salt and pepper, to taste

Instructions:

1. Heat olive oil in a large pot over medium heat. Add diced onion and garlic, and sauté for 3-4 minutes until softened.

2. Add the ground turkey and cook for 5-7 minutes, breaking it up with a spoon, until browned and fully cooked.

3. Stir in chili powder, cumin, smoked paprika, salt, and pepper. Add the diced tomatoes, black beans, kidney beans, and pinto beans.

4. Bring to a simmer and cook for 20 minutes, stirring occasionally.

5. Adjust seasoning to taste and serve hot.

Nutritional Value:
Calories 380 | Fat 10g | Saturated Fat 2g | Cholesterol 60mg | Sodium 450mg | Carbohydrate 47g | Fiber 15g | Added Sugar 0g | Protein 30g | Calcium 70mg | Potassium 900mg | Iron 4mg | Vitamin D 0mcg

Grilled Salmon with Lentil Salad

Prep Time: 15 minutes | **Cooking Time**: 20 minutes | **Total Time**: 35 minutes | **Serving**: 2 | **Cooking Difficulty**: Moderate

Ingredients:

- 2 salmon fillets (4-6 ounces each)

- 1 cup cooked lentils

- 1/2 cup cherry tomatoes, halved

- 1/4 red onion, finely chopped

- 1/4 cup fresh parsley, chopped

- 1 tablespoon olive oil (plus extra for grilling)

- 1 tablespoon lemon juice

- Salt and pepper, to taste

- 1/4 teaspoon garlic powder

Instructions:

1. Preheat the grill to medium heat.

2. Season the salmon fillets with olive oil, salt, pepper, and garlic powder. Grill the salmon for 4-5 minutes on each side until fully cooked.

3. In a mixing bowl, combine the cooked lentils, cherry tomatoes, red onion, and parsley.

4. Drizzle the lentil salad with olive oil and lemon juice, then toss to combine. Season with salt and pepper to taste.

5. Serve the grilled salmon on top of the lentil salad.

Nutritional Value:
Calories 400 | Fat 18g | Saturated Fat 3g | Cholesterol 70mg | Sodium 250mg | Carbohydrate 26g | Fiber 9g | Added Sugar 0g | Protein 36g | Calcium 60mg | Potassium 750mg | Iron 4mg | Vitamin D 10mcg

Turkey and White Bean Stew

Prep Time: 10 minutes | **Cooking Time**: 30 minutes | **Total Time**: 40 minutes | **Serving**: 4 | **Cooking Difficulty**: Easy

Ingredients:

- 1 pound ground turkey

- 1 can (15 ounces) white beans, drained and rinsed

- 1 onion, diced

- 2 carrots, diced

- 2 celery stalks, diced

- 1 can (14 ounces) diced tomatoes

- 4 cups chicken broth (low sodium)

- 2 cloves garlic, minced

- 1 teaspoon thyme

- 1/2 teaspoon paprika

- 1 tablespoon olive oil

- Salt and pepper, to taste

Instructions:

1. Heat olive oil in a large pot over medium heat. Add diced onion, garlic, carrots, and celery, and sauté for 5 minutes until softened.

2. Add the ground turkey and cook for 6-8 minutes until browned and fully cooked.

3. Stir in thyme, paprika, salt, and pepper. Add the diced tomatoes, white beans, and chicken broth.

4. Bring the stew to a simmer and cook for 20 minutes until vegetables are tender.

5. Adjust seasoning and serve hot.

Nutritional Value:
Calories 310 | Fat 10g | Saturated Fat 2g | Cholesterol 55mg | Sodium 500mg | Carbohydrate 32g | Fiber 10g | Added Sugar 0g | Protein 28g | Calcium 80mg | Potassium 900mg | Iron 4mg | Vitamin D 0mcg

Tempeh Taco Bowl

Prep Time: 10 minutes | **Cooking Time**: 15 minutes | **Total Time**: 25 minutes | **Serving**: 2 | **Cooking Difficulty**: Easy

Ingredients:

- 1 (8-ounce) block tempeh, crumbled

- 1/2 cup cooked quinoa

- 1/2 cup black beans, drained and rinsed

- 1/2 cup corn kernels (fresh or frozen)

- 1/4 cup salsa

- 1/2 teaspoon cumin

- 1/2 teaspoon chili powder

- 1 tablespoon olive oil
- Salt and pepper, to taste
- Avocado, for topping (optional)

Instructions:

1. Heat olive oil in a skillet over medium heat. Add the crumbled tempeh, cumin, chili powder, salt, and pepper. Cook for 5-7 minutes until browned and heated through.

2. In a bowl, layer the cooked quinoa, black beans, corn, and salsa.

3. Top the bowl with the cooked tempeh. Add avocado if desired.

4. Serve immediately.

Nutritional Value:

Calories 360 | Fat 15g | Saturated Fat 2g | Cholesterol 0mg | Sodium 280mg | Carbohydrate 40g | Fiber 10g | Added Sugar 0g | Protein 20g | Calcium 80mg | Potassium 600mg | Iron 3mg | Vitamin D 0mcg

Black Bean and Sweet Potato Enchiladas

Prep Time: 20 minutes | **Cooking Time:** 30 minutes | **Total Time:** 50 minutes | **Serving:** 4 | **Cooking Difficulty:** Moderate

Ingredients:

- 2 medium sweet potatoes, peeled and diced
- 1 can (15 ounces) black beans, drained and rinsed
- 8 small whole-wheat tortillas
- 1 cup enchilada sauce (store-bought or homemade)
- 1/2 cup shredded cheese (optional)
- 1/2 teaspoon cumin

- 1/4 teaspoon chili powder
- 1 tablespoon olive oil
- Salt and pepper, to taste

Instructions:

1. Preheat the oven to 375°F (190°C).

2. In a skillet, heat olive oil over medium heat. Add diced sweet potatoes, cumin, chili powder, salt, and pepper. Cook for 8-10 minutes until tender.

3. Stir in the black beans and cook for another 2 minutes.

4. Fill each tortilla with the sweet potato and black bean mixture, roll them up, and place them in a baking dish.

5. Pour the enchilada sauce over the rolled tortillas and top with shredded cheese if using.

6. Bake for 20 minutes until the cheese is melted and the enchiladas are heated through.

7. Serve warm.

Nutritional Value:

Calories 400 | Fat 10g | Saturated Fat 3g | Cholesterol 10mg | Sodium 550mg | Carbohydrate 62g | Fiber 14g | Added Sugar 0g | Protein 12g | Calcium 200mg | Potassium 900mg | Iron 4mg | Vitamin D 0mcg

Tofu and Edamame Stir-Fry

Prep Time: 10 minutes | **Cooking Time**: 15 minutes | **Total Time**: 25 minutes | **Serving**: 2 | **Cooking Difficulty**: Easy

Ingredients:

- 1 (14-ounce) block tofu, pressed and cubed
- 1/2 cup shelled edamame
- 1 bell pepper, sliced
- 1 tablespoon soy sauce (low sodium)
- 1 tablespoon sesame oil
- 1 clove garlic, minced
- 1 teaspoon ginger, minced
- 1 tablespoon sesame seeds (optional)
- Salt and pepper, to taste

Instructions:

1. Heat sesame oil in a skillet or wok over medium heat. Add cubed tofu and cook for 5-7 minutes until golden brown on all sides.
2. Add the garlic, ginger, bell pepper, and edamame. Stir-fry for 5 minutes until the vegetables are tender.
3. Stir in the soy sauce and cook for another 2 minutes.
4. Sprinkle with sesame seeds if desired. Serve warm.

Nutritional Value:
Calories 340 | Fat 18g | Saturated Fat 3g | Cholesterol 0mg | Sodium 400mg | Carbohydrate 22g | Fiber 6g | Added Sugar 0g | Protein 28g | Calcium 300mg | Potassium 450mg | Iron 4mg | Vitamin D 0mcg

Baked Cod with Black-Eyed Peas

Prep Time: 10 minutes | **Cooking Time**: 25 minutes | **Total Time**: 35 minutes | **Serving**: 2 | **Cooking Difficulty**: Easy

Ingredients:

- 2 cod fillets (4-6 ounces each)
- 1 cup cooked black-eyed peas (or 1 can, drained and rinsed)
- 1/2 cup diced tomatoes
- 1/4 red onion, finely chopped
- 2 cloves garlic, minced
- 1 tablespoon olive oil
- 1 teaspoon paprika
- 1/2 teaspoon cumin
- 1 tablespoon lemon juice
- Salt and pepper, to taste
- Fresh parsley, for garnish

Instructions:

1. Preheat the oven to 375°F (190°C).
2. Season the cod fillets with olive oil, paprika, cumin, salt, and pepper. Place them in a baking dish.
3. In a bowl, mix the black-eyed peas, diced tomatoes, red onion, garlic, and lemon juice. Spoon this mixture around the cod fillets.
4. Bake for 20-25 minutes until the cod is cooked through and flakes easily with a fork.
5. Garnish with fresh parsley and serve.

Nutritional Value:
Calories 320 | Fat 10g | Saturated Fat 2g | Cholesterol 60mg | Sodium 300mg | Carbohydrate 24g | Fiber 7g |

Added Sugar 0g | Protein 35g | Calcium 60mg | Potassium 700mg | Iron 2.5mg | Vitamin D 1.5mcg

Chicken and Chickpea Tagine

Prep Time: 15 minutes | **Cooking Time**: 40 minutes | **Total Time**: 55 minutes | **Serving**: 4 | **Cooking Difficulty**: Moderate

Ingredients:

- 1 pound chicken thighs, boneless and skinless
- 1 can (15 ounces) chickpeas, drained and rinsed
- 1 onion, diced
- 2 cloves garlic, minced
- 1/2 teaspoon ground cinnamon
- 1/2 teaspoon cumin
- 1/4 teaspoon turmeric
- 1 cup chicken broth (low sodium)
- 1/2 cup diced tomatoes
- 1/4 cup dried apricots, chopped
- 1 tablespoon olive oil
- Salt and pepper, to taste
- Fresh cilantro, for garnish

Instructions:

1. Heat olive oil in a large skillet over medium heat. Add the diced onion and garlic, and sauté for 5 minutes until softened.

2. Season the chicken thighs with cinnamon, cumin, turmeric, salt, and pepper. Add to the skillet and brown for 5-7 minutes on each side.

3. Stir in the chickpeas, diced tomatoes, apricots, and chicken broth. Bring to a simmer and cover the skillet. Cook for 25-30 minutes until the chicken is fully cooked and the flavors meld.

4. Garnish with fresh cilantro and serve over couscous or rice.

Nutritional Value:

Calories 420 | Fat 18g | Saturated Fat 4g | Cholesterol 85mg | Sodium 380mg | Carbohydrate 38g | Fiber 8g | Added Sugar 0g | Protein 30g | Calcium 80mg | Potassium 800mg | Iron 3mg | Vitamin D 0mcg

Seitan and Navy Bean Stew

Prep Time: 10 minutes | **Cooking Time**: 25 minutes | **Total Time**: 35 minutes | **Serving**: 4 | **Cooking Difficulty**: Moderate

Ingredients:

- 1 cup seitan, cubed
- 1 can (15 ounces) navy beans, drained and rinsed
- 1 carrot, diced
- 1 celery stalk, diced
- 1 small onion, diced
- 2 cloves garlic, minced
- 2 cups vegetable broth (low sodium)
- 1/2 teaspoon thyme
- 1/4 teaspoon smoked paprika
- 1 tablespoon olive oil
- Salt and pepper, to taste

Instructions:

1. Heat olive oil in a large pot over medium heat. Add the onion, carrot, celery, and garlic. Sauté for 5-7 minutes until softened.

2. Add the cubed seitan and cook for 3-4 minutes until lightly browned.

3. Stir in the navy beans, vegetable broth, thyme, paprika, salt, and pepper.

4. Bring the stew to a simmer and cook for 20 minutes until the flavors meld and the vegetables are tender.

5. Serve warm with crusty bread.

Nutritional Value:
Calories 280 | Fat 9g | Saturated Fat 1.5g | Cholesterol 0mg | Sodium 400mg | Carbohydrate 30g | Fiber 8g | Added Sugar 0g | Protein 22g | Calcium 90mg | Potassium 500mg | Iron 4mg | Vitamin D 0mcg

Tuna and Cannellini Bean Salad

Prep Time: 10 minutes | **Cooking Time**: 0 minutes | **Total Time**: 10 minutes | **Serving**: 2 | **Cooking Difficulty**: Easy

Ingredients:

- 1 can (5 ounces) tuna in water, drained
- 1 can (15 ounces) cannellini beans, drained and rinsed
- 1/4 red onion, finely chopped
- 1/4 cup fresh parsley, chopped
- 1 tablespoon capers (optional)
- 1 tablespoon lemon juice
- 2 tablespoons olive oil
- Salt and pepper, to taste

Instructions:

1. In a large bowl, combine the tuna, cannellini beans, red onion, parsley, and capers if using.

2. Drizzle with olive oil and lemon juice. Season with salt and pepper to taste.

3. Toss until well combined. Serve immediately or refrigerate for up to 2 days.

Nutritional Value:
Calories 320 | Fat 14g | Saturated Fat 2g | Cholesterol 25mg | Sodium 450mg | Carbohydrate 25g | Fiber 8g | Added Sugar 0g | Protein 28g | Calcium 90mg | Potassium 600mg | Iron 3mg | Vitamin D 0mcg

Bison and Kidney Bean Chili

Prep Time: 15 minutes | **Cooking Time**: 45 minutes | **Total Time**: 1 hour | **Serving**: 4 | **Cooking Difficulty**: Moderate

Ingredients:

- 1 pound ground bison
- 1 can (15 ounces) kidney beans, drained and rinsed
- 1 can (14 ounces) diced tomatoes
- 1 onion, diced
- 2 cloves garlic, minced
- 1 tablespoon chili powder
- 1 teaspoon cumin
- 1/2 teaspoon smoked paprika
- 1 tablespoon olive oil
- Salt and pepper, to taste
- Fresh cilantro, for garnish (optional)

Instructions:

1. Heat olive oil in a large pot over medium heat. Add the diced onion and garlic, and sauté for 5 minutes until softened.

2. Add the ground bison and cook for 7-10 minutes until browned and fully cooked.

3. Stir in the chili powder, cumin, paprika, salt, and pepper. Add the diced tomatoes and kidney beans.

4. Bring the chili to a simmer and cook for 30 minutes, stirring occasionally.

5. Garnish with fresh cilantro and serve hot.

Nutritional Value:
Calories 410 | Fat 18g | Saturated Fat 6g | Cholesterol 75mg | Sodium 480mg | Carbohydrate 32g | Fiber 10g | Added Sugar 0g | Protein 32g | Calcium 80mg | Potassium 800mg | Iron 4mg | Vitamin D 0mcg

Shrimp and Edamame Quinoa Bowl

Prep Time: 10 minutes | **Cooking Time:** 20 minutes | **Total Time:** 30 minutes | **Serving:** 2 | **Cooking Difficulty:** Easy

Ingredients:

- 1/2 pound shrimp, peeled and deveined
- 1/2 cup quinoa, rinsed
- 1 cup water or vegetable broth
- 1/2 cup shelled edamame
- 1/2 avocado, sliced
- 1 tablespoon soy sauce (low sodium)
- 1 tablespoon sesame oil
- 1 clove garlic, minced
- 1 tablespoon sesame seeds (optional)
- Salt and pepper, to taste

Instructions:

1. Cook quinoa in water or vegetable broth according to package instructions. Set aside.

2. Heat sesame oil in a skillet over medium heat. Add the minced garlic and shrimp. Cook for 3-4 minutes until shrimp are pink and fully cooked.

3. In the same skillet, add the edamame and cook for an additional 2 minutes. Season with soy sauce, salt, and pepper.

4. Divide the quinoa between two bowls and top with the shrimp, edamame, and avocado slices.

5. Sprinkle with sesame seeds if desired and serve warm.

Nutritional Value:
Calories 390 | Fat 18g | Saturated Fat 3g | Cholesterol 150mg | Sodium 620mg | Carbohydrate 30g | Fiber 8g | Added Sugar 0g | Protein 30g | Calcium 90mg | Potassium 700mg | Iron 3mg | Vitamin D 0mcg

Moroccan Lentil Meatballs

Prep Time: 15 minutes | **Cooking Time:** 25 minutes | **Total Time:** 40 minutes | **Serving:** 4 | **Cooking Difficulty:** Moderate

Ingredients:

- 1 cup cooked lentils
- 1/4 cup breadcrumbs (whole wheat or gluten-free)
- 1 egg (or flax egg for vegan)
- 1/4 cup chopped parsley
- 1/2 teaspoon cumin
- 1/2 teaspoon ground coriander
- 1/4 teaspoon cinnamon
- 1 tablespoon olive oil (for frying)
- Salt and pepper, to taste
- 1 cup tomato sauce (for serving)

Instructions:

1. In a large mixing bowl, combine cooked lentils, breadcrumbs, egg, parsley, cumin, coriander, cinnamon, salt, and pepper. Mix until well combined.

2. Form the mixture into small meatballs (about 12).

3. Heat olive oil in a skillet over medium heat. Fry the lentil meatballs for 3-4 minutes on each side until golden brown.

4. Serve with warm tomato sauce and garnish with extra parsley.

Nutritional Value:

Calories 250 | Fat 9g | Saturated Fat 1.5g | Cholesterol 35mg | Sodium 320mg | Carbohydrate 32g | Fiber 8g | Added Sugar 0g | Protein 12g | Calcium 60mg | Potassium 500mg | Iron 3mg | Vitamin D 0mcg

Turkey and Black Bean Stuffed Peppers

Prep Time: 15 minutes | **Cooking Time**: 30 minutes | **Total Time**: 45 minutes | **Serving**: 4 | **Cooking Difficulty**: Moderate

Ingredients:

- 4 large bell peppers, tops removed and seeds discarded
- 1/2 pound ground turkey
- 1 can (15 ounces) black beans, drained and rinsed
- 1/2 cup cooked quinoa
- 1/2 cup diced tomatoes
- 1/2 onion, diced
- 1 teaspoon cumin
- 1 teaspoon chili powder
- 1 tablespoon olive oil
- Salt and pepper, to taste
- 1/4 cup shredded cheese (optional)

Instructions:

1. Preheat the oven to 375°F (190°C).

2. Heat olive oil in a skillet over medium heat. Add diced onion and ground turkey. Cook for 6-8 minutes until turkey is browned.

3. Stir in the black beans, cooked quinoa, diced tomatoes, cumin, chili powder, salt, and pepper. Cook for an additional 3-4 minutes until heated through.

4. Stuff each bell pepper with the turkey and black bean mixture. Place them in a baking dish.

5. Bake for 25-30 minutes until the peppers are tender. If using cheese, sprinkle it on top of the peppers during the last 5 minutes of baking.

6. Serve warm.

Nutritional Value:

Calories 330 | Fat 12g | Saturated Fat 3g | Cholesterol 55mg | Sodium 420mg | Carbohydrate 35g | Fiber 10g | Added Sugar 0g | Protein 22g | Calcium 90mg | Potassium 900mg | Iron 3mg | Vitamin D 0mcg

Tofu and Mung Bean Curry

Prep Time: 10 minutes | **Cooking Time**: 30 minutes | **Total Time**: 40 minutes | **Serving**: 4 | **Cooking Difficulty**: Moderate

Ingredients:

- 1 block (14 ounces) tofu, pressed and cubed
- 1 cup cooked mung beans
- 1 onion, diced
- 2 cloves garlic, minced
- 1 tablespoon curry powder
- 1/2 teaspoon turmeric
- 1 can (14 ounces) coconut milk
- 1/2 cup diced tomatoes
- 1 tablespoon olive oil
- Salt and pepper, to taste

- Fresh cilantro, for garnish (optional)

Instructions:

1. Heat olive oil in a large skillet over medium heat. Add diced onion and garlic, and sauté for 5 minutes until softened.

2. Stir in the curry powder and turmeric, and cook for 1 minute until fragrant.

3. Add cubed tofu, cooked mung beans, coconut milk, and diced tomatoes. Bring to a simmer and cook for 20-25 minutes until the sauce thickens.

4. Season with salt and pepper to taste. Garnish with fresh cilantro and serve over rice or quinoa.

Nutritional Value:

Calories 380 | Fat 22g | Saturated Fat 10g | Cholesterol 0mg | Sodium 320mg | Carbohydrate 26g | Fiber 8g | Added Sugar 0g | Protein 20g | Calcium 150mg | Potassium 650mg | Iron 4mg | Vitamin D 0mcg

Lamb and Lima Bean Stew

Prep Time: 15 minutes | **Cooking Time**: 1 hour | **Total Time**: 1 hour 15 minutes | **Serving**: 4 | **Cooking Difficulty**: Moderate

Ingredients:

- 1 pound lamb stew meat, cubed

- 1 cup dried lima beans, soaked overnight and drained

- 1 onion, diced

- 2 carrots, diced

- 2 cloves garlic, minced

- 1 teaspoon thyme

- 1/2 teaspoon cumin

- 4 cups beef broth (low sodium)

- 1 tablespoon olive oil

- Salt and pepper, to taste

Instructions:

1. Heat olive oil in a large pot over medium heat. Add the lamb and brown for 5-7 minutes on all sides.

2. Add the diced onion, carrots, and garlic to the pot. Cook for 5 minutes until the vegetables soften.

3. Stir in the thyme, cumin, salt, and pepper. Add the lima beans and beef broth.

4. Bring the stew to a boil, then reduce the heat to low. Cover and simmer for 1 hour until the lamb is tender and the lima beans are fully cooked.

5. Adjust seasoning to taste and serve warm.

Nutritional Value:

Calories 450 | Fat 20g | Saturated Fat 7g | Cholesterol 90mg | Sodium 500mg | Carbohydrate 30g | Fiber 9g | Added Sugar 0g | Protein 35g | Calcium 70mg | Potassium 850mg | Iron 5mg | Vitamin D 0mcg

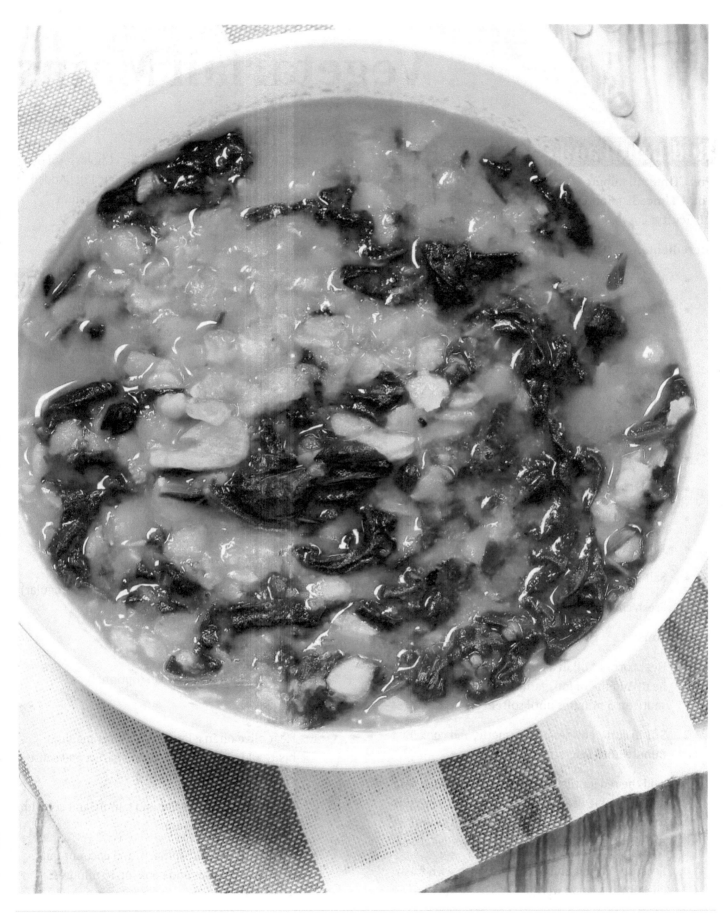

Vegetarian Mains

Red Lentil and Cauliflower Dal

Prep Time: 10 minutes | **Cooking Time**: 25 minutes | **Total Time**: 35 minutes | **Serving**: 4 | **Cooking Difficulty**: Easy

Ingredients:

- 1 cup red lentils, rinsed
- 1/2 head cauliflower, cut into small florets
- 1 onion, diced
- 2 cloves garlic, minced
- 1 tablespoon ginger, minced
- 1 tablespoon curry powder
- 1/2 teaspoon turmeric
- 1 can (14 ounces) diced tomatoes
- 2 cups vegetable broth (low sodium)
- 1 tablespoon coconut oil
- Salt and pepper, to taste
- Fresh cilantro, for garnish (optional)

Instructions:

1. Heat coconut oil in a large pot over medium heat. Add the onion, garlic, and ginger, and sauté for 5 minutes until softened.
2. Stir in curry powder and turmeric, and cook for 1 minute until fragrant.
3. Add the red lentils, cauliflower, diced tomatoes, and vegetable broth. Bring to a simmer and cook for 20-25 minutes, stirring occasionally, until the lentils are soft and the cauliflower is tender.
4. Season with salt and pepper. Garnish with fresh cilantro and serve warm.

Nutritional Value:
Calories 280 | Fat 6g | Saturated Fat 3g | Cholesterol 0mg | Sodium 320mg | Carbohydrate 45g | Fiber 12g | Added Sugar 0g | Protein 15g | Calcium 80mg | Potassium 850mg | Iron 5mg | Vitamin D 0mcg

Chickpea and Spinach Curry

Prep Time: 10 minutes | **Cooking Time**: 20 minutes | **Total Time**: 30 minutes | **Serving**: 4 | **Cooking Difficulty**: Easy

Ingredients:

- 1 can (15 ounces) chickpeas, drained and rinsed
- 4 cups fresh spinach
- 1 onion, diced
- 2 cloves garlic, minced
- 1 tablespoon curry powder
- 1 teaspoon ground cumin
- 1 can (14 ounces) coconut milk (light or regular)
- 1 tablespoon olive oil
- Salt and pepper, to taste
- Fresh cilantro, for garnish (optional)

Instructions:

1. Heat olive oil in a large skillet over medium heat. Add the diced onion and garlic, and sauté for 5 minutes until softened.
2. Stir in the curry powder and cumin, and cook for 1 minute until fragrant.
3. Add the chickpeas, spinach, and coconut milk. Bring to a simmer and cook for 10 minutes,

stirring occasionally, until the spinach wilts and the sauce thickens.

4. Season with salt and pepper. Garnish with fresh cilantro and serve with rice or naan.

Nutritional Value:
Calories 300 | Fat 18g | Saturated Fat 10g | Cholesterol 0mg | Sodium 380mg | Carbohydrate 28g | Fiber 8g | Added Sugar 0g | Protein 10g | Calcium 100mg | Potassium 700mg | Iron 4mg | Vitamin D 0mcg

Three Bean Veggie Burgers

Prep Time: 15 minutes | **Cooking Time:** 15 minutes | **Total Time:** 30 minutes | **Serving:** 4 | **Cooking Difficulty:** Moderate

Ingredients:

- 1/2 cup black beans, drained and rinsed
- 1/2 cup kidney beans, drained and rinsed
- 1/2 cup chickpeas, drained and rinsed
- 1/4 cup breadcrumbs (whole wheat or gluten-free)
- 1/4 cup diced onion
- 1 clove garlic, minced
- 1 teaspoon cumin
- 1/2 teaspoon smoked paprika
- 1 tablespoon olive oil (for cooking)
- Salt and pepper, to taste

Instructions:

1. In a large bowl, mash the black beans, kidney beans, and chickpeas until mostly smooth.

2. Stir in the breadcrumbs, diced onion, garlic, cumin, smoked paprika, salt, and pepper. Mix until well combined.

3. Form the mixture into 4 patties.

4. Heat olive oil in a skillet over medium heat. Cook the patties for 4-5 minutes on each side until golden brown and heated through.

5. Serve on whole-grain buns or lettuce wraps with your favorite toppings.

Nutritional Value:
Calories 300 | Fat 10g | Saturated Fat 1.5g | Cholesterol 0mg | Sodium 350mg | Carbohydrate 45g | Fiber 12g | Added Sugar 0g | Protein 14g | Calcium 90mg | Potassium 650mg | Iron 3.5mg | Vitamin D 0mcg

Tempeh and Black Bean Tacos

Prep Time: 10 minutes | **Cooking Time:** 15 minutes | **Total Time:** 25 minutes | **Serving:** 4 | **Cooking Difficulty:** Easy

Ingredients:

- 1 block (8 ounces) tempeh, crumbled
- 1 can (15 ounces) black beans, drained and rinsed
- 1/2 teaspoon cumin
- 1/2 teaspoon chili powder
- 1/4 cup salsa
- 1 tablespoon olive oil
- 8 small corn tortillas
- Toppings: avocado, shredded lettuce, chopped tomatoes, cheese (optional)

Instructions:

1. Heat olive oil in a skillet over medium heat. Add crumbled tempeh, cumin, and chili powder, and cook for 5-7 minutes until the tempeh is browned.

2. Stir in the black beans and salsa, and cook for an additional 2-3 minutes until heated through.

3. Warm the corn tortillas in a dry skillet or microwave.

4. Divide the tempeh and black bean mixture among the tortillas and top with avocado, lettuce, tomatoes, and cheese if desired.

5. Serve immediately.

Nutritional Value:

Calories 320 | Fat 12g | Saturated Fat 2g | Cholesterol 0mg | Sodium 420mg | Carbohydrate 40g | Fiber 12g | Added Sugar 0g | Protein 18g | Calcium 80mg | Potassium 600mg | Iron 3mg | Vitamin D 0mcg

Quinoa-Stuffed Eggplant

Prep Time: 15 minutes | **Cooking Time:** 35 minutes | **Total Time:** 50 minutes | **Serving:** 4 | **Cooking Difficulty:** Moderate

Ingredients:

- 2 medium eggplants, halved lengthwise
- 1 cup cooked quinoa
- 1/2 cup diced tomatoes
- 1/4 cup feta cheese (optional)
- 1/4 cup fresh parsley, chopped
- 1 tablespoon olive oil
- 1 teaspoon oregano
- Salt and pepper, to taste

Instructions:

1. Preheat the oven to 375°F (190°C).

2. Scoop out the flesh of the eggplants, leaving a 1/2-inch border around the edges. Chop the eggplant flesh and set aside.

3. Place the eggplant halves in a baking dish, drizzle with olive oil, and bake for 20 minutes until softened.

4. Meanwhile, in a skillet, cook the chopped eggplant flesh with oregano, salt, and pepper for

5 minutes. Stir in the cooked quinoa and diced tomatoes, and cook for another 5 minutes.

5. Remove the eggplant halves from the oven and stuff them with the quinoa mixture. Top with feta cheese if using.

6. Bake for an additional 10-15 minutes until heated through.

7. Garnish with fresh parsley and serve.

Nutritional Value:

Calories 280 | Fat 10g | Saturated Fat 2g | Cholesterol 10mg | Sodium 320mg | Carbohydrate 40g | Fiber 10g | Added Sugar 0g | Protein 8g | Calcium 120mg | Potassium 650mg | Iron 2.5mg | Vitamin D 0mcg

Bean and Barley Buddha Bowl

Prep Time: 15 minutes | **Cooking Time:** 25 minutes | **Total Time:** 40 minutes | **Serving:** 2 | **Cooking Difficulty:** Easy

Ingredients:

- 1/2 cup cooked barley
- 1/2 cup black beans, drained and rinsed
- 1/2 cup chickpeas, drained and rinsed
- 1/2 avocado, sliced
- 1/4 cup shredded carrots
- 1/4 cup cucumber slices
- 1 tablespoon olive oil
- 1 tablespoon lemon juice
- Salt and pepper, to taste
- Sesame seeds, for garnish (optional)

Instructions:

1. In two serving bowls, layer the cooked barley, black beans, chickpeas, avocado slices, shredded carrots, and cucumber slices.

2. In a small bowl, whisk together olive oil, lemon juice, salt, and pepper.

3. Drizzle the dressing over the Buddha bowls and garnish with sesame seeds if desired.

4. Serve immediately.

Nutritional Value:

Calories 380 | Fat 14g | Saturated Fat 2g | Cholesterol 0mg | Sodium 250mg | Carbohydrate 52g | Fiber 12g | Added Sugar 0g | Protein 12g | Calcium 70mg | Potassium 800mg | Iron 3mg | Vitamin D 0mcg

Lentil Shepherd's Pie

Prep Time: 20 minutes | **Cooking Time:** 35 minutes | **Total Time:** 55 minutes | **Serving:** 4 | **Cooking Difficulty:** Moderate

Ingredients:

- 1 cup cooked lentils

- 2 cups mashed potatoes

- 1 onion, diced

- 2 carrots, diced

- 1 cup green peas (fresh or frozen)

- 1 tablespoon olive oil

- 1 teaspoon thyme

- 1/2 teaspoon smoked paprika

- Salt and pepper, to taste

Instructions:

1. Preheat the oven to 375°F (190°C).

2. Heat olive oil in a skillet over medium heat. Add the diced onion and carrots, and sauté for 5-7 minutes until softened.

3. Stir in the cooked lentils, green peas, thyme, smoked paprika, salt, and pepper. Cook for an additional 5 minutes.

4. Transfer the lentil mixture to a baking dish and spread the mashed potatoes on top.

5. Bake for 20-25 minutes until the top is golden brown.

6. Serve warm.

Nutritional Value:

Calories 320 | Fat 7g | Saturated Fat 1.5g | Cholesterol 0mg | Sodium 300mg | Carbohydrate 55g | Fiber 12g | Added Sugar 0g | Protein 12g | Calcium 80mg | Potassium 800mg | Iron 4mg | Vitamin D 0mcg

Tofu and Edamame Noodle Bowl

Prep Time: 10 minutes | **Cooking Time:** 15 minutes | **Total Time:** 25 minutes | **Serving:** 2 | **Cooking Difficulty:** Easy

Ingredients:

- 1 block (14 ounces) tofu, cubed

- 1/2 cup shelled edamame

- 4 ounces rice noodles

- 1 tablespoon soy sauce (low sodium)

- 1 tablespoon sesame oil

- 1 clove garlic, minced

- 1/2 teaspoon ginger, minced

- 1 tablespoon sesame seeds (optional)

- 2 green onions, sliced (optional)

Instructions:

1. Cook rice noodles according to package instructions. Drain and set aside.

2. In a skillet, heat sesame oil over medium heat. Add cubed tofu, garlic, and ginger. Cook for 5-7 minutes until the tofu is golden brown on all sides.

3. Stir in the shelled edamame and soy sauce. Cook for another 2-3 minutes.

4. Divide the cooked noodles between two bowls and top with the tofu and edamame mixture.

5. Garnish with sesame seeds and sliced green onions if desired. Serve warm.

Nutritional Value:

Calories 400 | Fat 18g | Saturated Fat 3g | Cholesterol 0mg | Sodium 450mg | Carbohydrate 40g | Fiber 6g | Added Sugar 0g | Protein 25g | Calcium 250mg | Potassium 600mg | Iron 4mg | Vitamin D 0mcg

Black Bean and Sweet Potato Patties

Prep Time: 15 minutes | **Cooking Time**: 20 minutes | **Total Time**: 35 minutes | **Serving**: 4 | **Cooking Difficulty**: Moderate

Ingredients:

- 1 can (15 ounces) black beans, drained and rinsed

- 1 cup mashed sweet potato

- 1/4 cup breadcrumbs (whole wheat or gluten-free)

- 1/2 teaspoon cumin

- 1/2 teaspoon smoked paprika

- 1 tablespoon olive oil (for frying)

- Salt and pepper, to taste

Instructions:

1. In a large bowl, mash the black beans with a fork or potato masher until mostly smooth.

2. Stir in the mashed sweet potato, breadcrumbs, cumin, smoked paprika, salt, and pepper. Mix until well combined.

3. Form the mixture into 4 patties.

4. Heat olive oil in a skillet over medium heat. Cook the patties for 4-5 minutes on each side until golden brown and heated through.

5. Serve on buns or with a side salad.

Nutritional Value:

Calories 290 | Fat 8g | Saturated Fat 1.5g | Cholesterol 0mg | Sodium 350mg | Carbohydrate 48g | Fiber 12g | Added Sugar 0g | Protein 10g | Calcium 80mg | Potassium 700mg | Iron 3mg | Vitamin D 0mcg

Split Pea and Mushroom Loaf

Prep Time: 15 minutes | **Cooking Time**: 45 minutes | **Total Time**: 1 hour | **Serving**: 4 | **Cooking Difficulty**: Moderate

Ingredients:

- 1 cup cooked split peas
- 1/2 cup chopped mushrooms
- 1/4 cup breadcrumbs (whole wheat or gluten-free)
- 1/4 cup chopped onion
- 1 clove garlic, minced
- 1 tablespoon soy sauce (low sodium)
- 1 tablespoon olive oil
- 1/2 teaspoon thyme
- Salt and pepper, to taste

Instructions:

1. Preheat the oven to 350°F (180°C).
2. Heat olive oil in a skillet over medium heat. Add the chopped mushrooms, onion, and garlic, and sauté for 5-7 minutes until softened.
3. In a large bowl, combine the cooked split peas, sautéed mushrooms, breadcrumbs, soy sauce, thyme, salt, and pepper. Mix until well combined.
4. Transfer the mixture to a greased loaf pan and press it down evenly.
5. Bake for 40-45 minutes until firm and golden brown on top.
6. Let the loaf cool for 10 minutes before slicing. Serve warm.

Nutritional Value:

Calories 330 | Fat 10g | Saturated Fat 2g | Cholesterol 0mg | Sodium 480mg | Carbohydrate 45g | Fiber 12g | Added Sugar 0g | Protein 15g | Calcium 90mg | Potassium 600mg | Iron 4mg | Vitamin D 0mcg

Grilled Chicken and Lentil Salad

Prep Time: 10 minutes | **Cooking Time:** 20 minutes | **Total Time:** 30 minutes | **Serving:** 2 | **Cooking Difficulty:** Easy

Ingredients:

- 2 chicken breasts (4-6 ounces each)
- 1 cup cooked lentils
- 1/2 cup cherry tomatoes, halved
- 1/4 red onion, thinly sliced
- 1/4 cup fresh parsley, chopped
- 1 tablespoon olive oil (plus extra for grilling)
- 1 tablespoon lemon juice
- Salt and pepper, to taste

Instructions:

1. Preheat the grill to medium heat. Rub the chicken breasts with olive oil, salt, and pepper.
2. Grill the chicken for 6-8 minutes on each side until fully cooked.
3. In a large bowl, combine the cooked lentils, cherry tomatoes, red onion, and parsley.
4. In a small bowl, whisk together olive oil and lemon juice, then pour over the lentil salad. Toss until well combined.
5. Slice the grilled chicken and serve on top of the lentil salad.

Nutritional Value:

Calories 400 | Fat 14g | Saturated Fat 2.5g | Cholesterol 90mg | Sodium 300mg | Carbohydrate 25g | Fiber 10g | Added Sugar 0g | Protein 40g | Calcium 60mg | Potassium 800mg | Iron 4mg | Vitamin D 0mcg

Three Bean Power Bowl

Prep Time: 10 minutes | **Cooking Time:** 10 minutes | **Total Time:** 20 minutes | **Serving:** 2 | **Cooking Difficulty:** Easy

Ingredients:

- 1/2 cup black beans, drained and rinsed
- 1/2 cup kidney beans, drained and rinsed
- 1/2 cup chickpeas, drained and rinsed
- 1/2 avocado, sliced
- 1/4 cup shredded carrots
- 1/4 cup diced cucumber
- 1 tablespoon olive oil
- 1 tablespoon lemon juice
- Salt and pepper, to taste
- Fresh cilantro, for garnish (optional)

Instructions:

1. In a serving bowl, layer the black beans, kidney beans, chickpeas, avocado, carrots, and cucumber.
2. In a small bowl, whisk together olive oil, lemon juice, salt, and pepper. Drizzle over the bowl.
3. Toss lightly to combine and garnish with cilantro if desired. Serve immediately.

Nutritional Value:
Calories 420 | Fat 18g | Saturated Fat 2.5g | Cholesterol 0mg | Sodium 300mg | Carbohydrate 55g | Fiber 17g | Added Sugar 0g | Protein 15g | Calcium 100mg | Potassium 900mg | Iron 4.5mg | Vitamin D 0mcg

Nutritional Value:
Calories 340 | Fat 14g | Saturated Fat 2g | Cholesterol 0mg | Sodium 280mg | Carbohydrate 45g | Fiber 10g | Added Sugar 0g | Protein 10g | Calcium 80mg | Potassium 550mg | Iron 3mg | Vitamin D 0mcg

Quinoa Chickpea Tabbouleh

Prep Time: 10 minutes | **Cooking Time:** 15 minutes | **Total Time:** 25 minutes | **Serving:** 4 | **Cooking Difficulty:** Easy

Ingredients:

- 1/2 cup quinoa, rinsed
- 1 cup water
- 1 can (15 ounces) chickpeas, drained and rinsed
- 1/2 cucumber, diced
- 1/2 cup cherry tomatoes, halved
- 1/4 cup fresh parsley, chopped
- 1/4 cup fresh mint, chopped
- 2 tablespoons olive oil
- 2 tablespoons lemon juice
- Salt and pepper, to taste

Instructions:

1. In a medium saucepan, bring quinoa and water to a boil. Reduce heat, cover, and simmer for 12-15 minutes until water is absorbed and quinoa is cooked. Fluff with a fork and let cool slightly.

2. In a large bowl, combine the cooked quinoa, chickpeas, cucumber, cherry tomatoes, parsley, and mint.

3. In a small bowl, whisk together olive oil and lemon juice. Pour over the quinoa mixture and toss until well combined.

4. Season with salt and pepper. Serve chilled or at room temperature.

Tuna and White Bean Niçoise

Prep Time: 10 minutes | **Cooking Time:** 0 minutes | **Total Time:** 10 minutes | **Serving:** 2 | **Cooking Difficulty:** Easy

Ingredients:

- 1 can (5 ounces) tuna in water, drained
- 1/2 cup canned white beans, drained and rinsed
- 1/4 cup cherry tomatoes, halved
- 1/4 cup green beans, blanched
- 2 hard-boiled eggs, halved
- 1/4 cup Kalamata olives, pitted
- 2 tablespoons olive oil
- 1 tablespoon lemon juice
- Salt and pepper, to taste

Instructions:

1. In a large bowl, combine tuna, white beans, cherry tomatoes, green beans, and Kalamata olives.

2. Drizzle with olive oil and lemon juice. Toss lightly to combine.

3. Arrange hard-boiled eggs on top and season with salt and pepper.

4. Serve chilled or at room temperature.

Nutritional Value:
Calories 350 | Fat 20g | Saturated Fat 3.5g | Cholesterol 230mg | Sodium 400mg | Carbohydrate 20g | Fiber 6g | Added Sugar 0g | Protein 28g | Calcium 90mg | Potassium 550mg | Iron 2.5mg | Vitamin D 0mcg

Tempeh and Black Bean Taco Salad

Prep Time: 10 minutes | **Cooking Time:** 15 minutes | **Total Time:** 25 minutes | **Serving:** 2 | **Cooking Difficulty:** Easy

Ingredients:

- 1 block (8 ounces) tempeh, crumbled
- 1/2 cup black beans, drained and rinsed
- 1/4 teaspoon cumin
- 1/4 teaspoon chili powder
- 1 tablespoon olive oil
- 4 cups mixed greens
- 1/2 avocado, diced
- 1/4 cup cherry tomatoes, halved
- 2 tablespoons salsa
- 1 tablespoon lime juice
- Salt and pepper, to taste

Instructions:

1. Heat olive oil in a skillet over medium heat. Add crumbled tempeh, cumin, chili powder, salt, and pepper. Cook for 5-7 minutes until tempeh is browned.
2. Stir in the black beans and cook for another 2 minutes until heated through.
3. In a large bowl, combine the mixed greens, avocado, and cherry tomatoes.
4. Top the salad with the tempeh and black bean mixture. Drizzle with salsa and lime juice.
5. Toss lightly to combine and serve.

Nutritional Value:

Calories 400 | Fat 18g | Saturated Fat 3g | Cholesterol 0mg | Sodium 300mg | Carbohydrate 40g | Fiber 14g | Added Sugar 0g | Protein 20g | Calcium 100mg | Potassium 800mg | Iron 4mg | Vitamin D 0mcg

Edamame and Salmon Poke Bowl

Prep Time: 10 minutes | **Cooking Time:** 0 minutes | **Total Time:** 10 minutes | **Serving:** 2 | **Cooking Difficulty:** Easy

Ingredients:

- 1/2 pound sushi-grade salmon, diced
- 1/2 cup cooked edamame
- 1 cup cooked brown rice
- 1/2 avocado, sliced
- 1/4 cup cucumber, thinly sliced
- 2 tablespoons soy sauce (low sodium)
- 1 tablespoon sesame oil
- 1 teaspoon rice vinegar
- 1 teaspoon sesame seeds (optional)
- 1 green onion, sliced (optional)

Instructions:

1. In a small bowl, whisk together soy sauce, sesame oil, and rice vinegar. Set aside.
2. Divide the cooked brown rice between two bowls. Top with diced salmon, edamame, avocado, and cucumber slices.
3. Drizzle the soy sauce mixture over the bowls and garnish with sesame seeds and green onions if desired.
4. Serve immediately.

Nutritional Value:

Calories 400 | Fat 20g | Saturated Fat 3.5g | Cholesterol 60mg | Sodium 600mg | Carbohydrate 30g | Fiber 7g | Added Sugar 0g | Protein 28g | Calcium 70mg | Potassium 800mg | Iron 2.5mg | Vitamin D 5mcg

Chicken and Navy Bean Greek Salad

Prep Time: 10 minutes | **Cooking Time:** 10 minutes | **Total Time:** 20 minutes | **Serving:** 2 | **Cooking Difficulty:** Easy

Ingredients:

- 2 chicken breasts (4-6 ounces each)
- 1/2 cup canned navy beans, drained and rinsed
- 1/2 cucumber, diced
- 1/2 cup cherry tomatoes, halved
- 1/4 cup Kalamata olives, pitted
- 1/4 cup crumbled feta cheese
- 1 tablespoon olive oil (plus extra for grilling)
- 1 tablespoon lemon juice
- Salt and pepper, to taste
- Fresh parsley, for garnish (optional)

Instructions:

1. Preheat the grill to medium heat. Rub the chicken breasts with olive oil, salt, and pepper. Grill for 6-8 minutes on each side until fully cooked. Slice and set aside.

2. In a large bowl, combine navy beans, cucumber, cherry tomatoes, olives, and feta cheese.

3. In a small bowl, whisk together olive oil and lemon juice. Drizzle over the salad and toss to combine.

4. Top the salad with sliced grilled chicken and garnish with parsley if desired.

Nutritional Value:

Calories 420 | Fat 18g | Saturated Fat 5g | Cholesterol 90mg | Sodium 500mg | Carbohydrate 25g | Fiber 7g | Added Sugar 0g | Protein 40g | Calcium 150mg | Potassium 750mg | Iron 3mg | Vitamin D 0mcg

Lentil and Grilled Halloumi Bowl

Prep Time: 10 minutes | **Cooking Time:** 10 minutes | **Total Time:** 20 minutes | **Serving:** 2 | **Cooking Difficulty:** Moderate

Ingredients:

- 1 cup cooked lentils
- 4 ounces halloumi cheese, sliced
- 1/2 cup cherry tomatoes, halved
- 1/4 red onion, thinly sliced
- 1 tablespoon olive oil
- 1 tablespoon lemon juice
- Salt and pepper, to taste
- Fresh mint leaves, for garnish (optional)

Instructions:

1. Heat a non-stick skillet over medium heat. Grill the halloumi slices for 2-3 minutes on each side until golden brown.

2. In a bowl, combine cooked lentils, cherry tomatoes, and red onion.

3. In a small bowl, whisk together olive oil and lemon juice. Drizzle over the lentil mixture and toss to combine. Season with salt and pepper.

4. Top with grilled halloumi and garnish with fresh mint if desired. Serve warm.

Nutritional Value:

Calories 450 | Fat 25g | Saturated Fat 10g | Cholesterol 40mg | Sodium 600mg | Carbohydrate 35g | Fiber 8g | Added Sugar 0g | Protein 25g | Calcium 400mg | Potassium 500mg | Iron 4mg | Vitamin D 0mcg

Turkey and Garbanzo Mediterranean Salad

Prep Time: 10 minutes | **Cooking Time:** 10 minutes | **Total Time:** 20 minutes | **Serving:** 2 | **Cooking Difficulty:** Easy

Ingredients:

- 1/2 pound ground turkey
- 1 can (15 ounces) chickpeas, drained and rinsed
- 1/2 cucumber, diced
- 1/2 cup cherry tomatoes, halved
- 1/4 cup crumbled feta cheese
- 1 tablespoon olive oil
- 1 tablespoon lemon juice
- 1/2 teaspoon oregano
- Salt and pepper, to taste

Instructions:

1. Heat a skillet over medium heat and cook the ground turkey for 6-8 minutes until browned and fully cooked. Set aside.

2. In a large bowl, combine chickpeas, cucumber, cherry tomatoes, and feta cheese.

3. In a small bowl, whisk together olive oil, lemon juice, oregano, salt, and pepper.

4. Add the cooked turkey to the salad and drizzle with the dressing. Toss lightly to combine and serve immediately.

Nutritional Value:

Calories 440 | Fat 20g | Saturated Fat 6g | Cholesterol 80mg | Sodium 500mg | Carbohydrate 35g | Fiber 9g | Added Sugar 0g | Protein 35g | Calcium 150mg | Potassium 800mg | Iron 4mg | Vitamin D 0mcg

Tofu and Mung Bean Asian Slaw

Prep Time: 15 minutes | **Cooking Time:** 10 minutes | **Total Time:** 25 minutes | **Serving:** 2 | **Cooking Difficulty:** Moderate

Ingredients:

- 1 block (14 ounces) tofu, pressed and cubed
- 1/2 cup cooked mung beans
- 2 cups shredded cabbage
- 1 carrot, julienned
- 1 tablespoon soy sauce (low sodium)
- 1 tablespoon rice vinegar
- 1 tablespoon sesame oil
- 1 teaspoon ginger, minced
- 1 tablespoon sesame seeds (optional)

Instructions:

1. Heat sesame oil in a skillet over medium heat. Add cubed tofu and ginger. Cook for 5-7 minutes until tofu is golden brown on all sides.

2. In a large bowl, combine shredded cabbage, julienned carrot, and cooked mung beans.

3. In a small bowl, whisk together soy sauce and rice vinegar. Pour over the slaw and toss to combine.

4. Top the slaw with cooked tofu and sprinkle with sesame seeds if desired. Serve chilled or at room temperature.

Nutritional Value:

Calories 380 | Fat 18g | Saturated Fat 2.5g | Cholesterol 0mg | Sodium 450mg | Carbohydrate 30g | Fiber 8g | Added Sugar 0g | Protein 25g | Calcium 250mg | Potassium 700mg | Iron 4mg | Vitamin D 0mcg

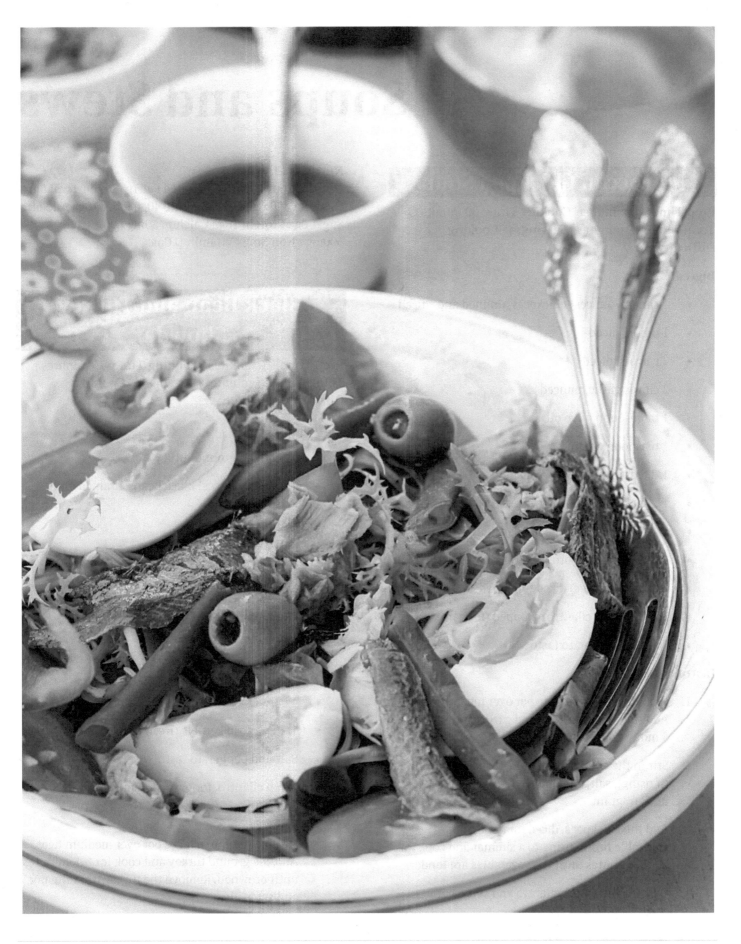

Soups and Stews

Moroccan Chickpea Soup

Prep Time: 10 minutes | **Cooking Time**: 30 minutes | **Total Time**: 40 minutes | **Serving**: 4 | **Cooking Difficulty**: Easy

Ingredients:

- 1 can (15 ounces) chickpeas, drained and rinsed
- 1 onion, diced
- 2 carrots, diced
- 2 cloves garlic, minced
- 1 tablespoon olive oil
- 1 teaspoon cumin
- 1/2 teaspoon ground cinnamon
- 1/2 teaspoon ground turmeric
- 1/4 teaspoon cayenne pepper (optional)
- 4 cups vegetable broth (low sodium)
- 1 can (14 ounces) diced tomatoes
- 1/4 cup fresh cilantro, chopped (for garnish)
- Salt and pepper, to taste

Instructions:

1. Heat olive oil in a large pot over medium heat. Add the onion, carrots, and garlic, and sauté for 5 minutes until softened.

2. Stir in the cumin, cinnamon, turmeric, cayenne (if using), salt, and pepper. Cook for 1 minute until fragrant.

3. Add the chickpeas, diced tomatoes, and vegetable broth. Bring to a simmer and cook for 20-25 minutes until the vegetables are tender.

4. Garnish with fresh cilantro and serve hot.

Nutritional Value:

Calories 260 | Fat 7g | Saturated Fat 1g | Cholesterol 0mg | Sodium 480mg | Carbohydrate 40g | Fiber 10g | Added Sugar 0g | Protein 10g | Calcium 80mg | Potassium 600mg | Iron 3mg | Vitamin D 0mcg

Black Bean and Turkey Chowder

Prep Time: 10 minutes | **Cooking Time**: 25 minutes | **Total Time**: 35 minutes | **Serving**: 4 | **Cooking Difficulty**: Moderate

Ingredients:

- 1/2 pound ground turkey
- 1 can (15 ounces) black beans, drained and rinsed
- 1 onion, diced
- 1 bell pepper, diced
- 2 cloves garlic, minced
- 1 tablespoon olive oil
- 1 teaspoon cumin
- 1/2 teaspoon smoked paprika
- 4 cups chicken broth (low sodium)
- 1/2 cup corn kernels (fresh or frozen)
- Salt and pepper, to taste
- Fresh cilantro, for garnish (optional)

Instructions:

1. Heat olive oil in a large pot over medium heat. Add the ground turkey and cook for 6-8 minutes until browned. Remove the turkey from the pot and set aside.

2. In the same pot, add the onion, bell pepper, and garlic, and sauté for 5 minutes until softened.

3. Stir in the cumin, smoked paprika, salt, and pepper. Add the black beans, chicken broth, and corn. Bring to a simmer and cook for 15 minutes.

4. Return the turkey to the pot and cook for an additional 5 minutes.

5. Garnish with fresh cilantro and serve hot.

Nutritional Value:
Calories 320 | Fat 10g | Saturated Fat 2g | Cholesterol 55mg | Sodium 550mg | Carbohydrate 35g | Fiber 10g | Added Sugar 0g | Protein 25g | Calcium 60mg | Potassium 700mg | Iron 3mg | Vitamin D 0mcg

Red Lentil and Quinoa Soup

Prep Time: 10 minutes | **Cooking Time**: 25 minutes | **Total Time**: 35 minutes | **Serving**: 4 | **Cooking Difficulty**: Easy

Ingredients:

- 1 cup red lentils, rinsed
- 1/4 cup quinoa, rinsed
- 1 onion, diced
- 2 cloves garlic, minced
- 1 tablespoon olive oil
- 1 teaspoon ground cumin
- 1/2 teaspoon turmeric
- 1/4 teaspoon smoked paprika
- 4 cups vegetable broth (low sodium)
- 1 can (14 ounces) diced tomatoes
- 1/4 cup fresh cilantro, chopped (for garnish)
- Salt and pepper, to taste

Instructions:

1. Heat olive oil in a large pot over medium heat. Add the onion and garlic, and sauté for 5 minutes until softened.

2. Stir in cumin, turmeric, smoked paprika, salt, and pepper. Cook for 1 minute until fragrant.

3. Add the red lentils, quinoa, diced tomatoes, and vegetable broth. Bring to a simmer and cook for 20-25 minutes until the lentils and quinoa are tender.

4. Garnish with fresh cilantro and serve hot.

Nutritional Value:
Calories 300 | Fat 8g | Saturated Fat 1g | Cholesterol 0mg | Sodium 460mg | Carbohydrate 45g | Fiber 10g | Added Sugar 0g | Protein 12g | Calcium 70mg | Potassium 650mg | Iron 3.5mg | Vitamin D 0mcg

Navy Bean and Chicken Stew

Prep Time: 10 minutes | **Cooking Time**: 30 minutes | **Total Time**: 40 minutes | **Serving**: 4 | **Cooking Difficulty**: Moderate

Ingredients:

- 1 pound boneless, skinless chicken thighs, diced
- 1 can (15 ounces) navy beans, drained and rinsed
- 1 onion, diced
- 2 carrots, diced
- 2 cloves garlic, minced
- 1 tablespoon olive oil
- 1 teaspoon thyme
- 4 cups chicken broth (low sodium)
- 1/2 cup diced tomatoes
- Salt and pepper, to taste

Instructions:

1. Heat olive oil in a large pot over medium heat. Add the diced chicken thighs and cook for 5-7 minutes until browned. Remove the chicken from the pot and set aside.

2. In the same pot, add the onion, carrots, and garlic, and sauté for 5 minutes until softened.

3. Stir in thyme, salt, and pepper. Add the navy beans, chicken broth, and diced tomatoes. Bring to a simmer and cook for 20 minutes.

4. Return the chicken to the pot and cook for an additional 10 minutes until fully cooked.

5. Serve hot.

Nutritional Value:
Calories 380 | Fat 12g | Saturated Fat 2.5g | Cholesterol 85mg | Sodium 480mg | Carbohydrate 35g | Fiber 9g | Added Sugar 0g | Protein 30g | Calcium 80mg | Potassium 750mg | Iron 4mg | Vitamin D 0mcg

Split Pea and Ham Hock Soup

Prep Time: 10 minutes | **Cooking Time**: 1 hour | **Total Time**: 1 hour 10 minutes | **Serving**: 4 | **Cooking Difficulty**: Moderate

Ingredients:

- 1 ham hock
- 1 cup dried split peas, rinsed
- 1 onion, diced
- 2 carrots, diced
- 2 cloves garlic, minced
- 1 teaspoon thyme
- 4 cups chicken broth (low sodium)
- 1 bay leaf
- Salt and pepper, to taste

Instructions:

1. In a large pot, combine the ham hock, split peas, onion, carrots, garlic, thyme, chicken broth, and bay leaf.

2. Bring the soup to a boil, then reduce the heat to low. Simmer for 1 hour, stirring occasionally, until the split peas are soft and the ham hock is tender.

3. Remove the ham hock and bay leaf from the soup. Shred the ham off the bone and return the meat to the soup.

4. Season with salt and pepper to taste. Serve hot.

Nutritional Value:
Calories 400 | Fat 14g | Saturated Fat 5g | Cholesterol 60mg | Sodium 650mg | Carbohydrate 40g | Fiber 13g | Added Sugar 0g | Protein 30g | Calcium 60mg | Potassium 700mg | Iron 4mg | Vitamin D 0mcg

Three Bean Vegetable Soup

Prep Time: 10 minutes | **Cooking Time**: 30 minutes | **Total Time**: 40 minutes | **Serving**: 4 | **Cooking Difficulty**: Easy

Ingredients:

- 1/2 cup black beans, drained and rinsed
- 1/2 cup kidney beans, drained and rinsed
- 1/2 cup chickpeas, drained and rinsed
- 1 onion, diced
- 2 carrots, diced
- 2 celery stalks, diced
- 2 cloves garlic, minced
- 1 can (14 ounces) diced tomatoes
- 4 cups vegetable broth (low sodium)
- 1 tablespoon olive oil
- 1 teaspoon thyme
- 1/2 teaspoon cumin
- Salt and pepper, to taste

Instructions:

1. Heat olive oil in a large pot over medium heat. Add the onion, carrots, celery, and garlic, and sauté for 5-7 minutes until softened.

2. Stir in thyme, cumin, salt, and pepper. Add the black beans, kidney beans, chickpeas, diced tomatoes, and vegetable broth.

3. Bring to a simmer and cook for 20-25 minutes until the vegetables are tender.

4. Adjust seasoning if needed. Serve hot.

Nutritional Value:
Calories 290 | Fat 6g | Saturated Fat 1g | Cholesterol 0mg | Sodium 460mg | Carbohydrate 45g | Fiber 12g | Added Sugar 0g | Protein 12g | Calcium 80mg | Potassium 650mg | Iron 3.5mg | Vitamin D 0mcg

Lentil and Barley Minestrone

Prep Time: 10 minutes | **Cooking Time**: 40 minutes | **Total Time**: 50 minutes | **Serving**: 4 | **Cooking Difficulty**: Moderate

Ingredients:

- 1/2 cup lentils, rinsed
- 1/2 cup pearl barley
- 1 onion, diced
- 2 carrots, diced
- 2 celery stalks, diced
- 2 cloves garlic, minced
- 1 can (14 ounces) diced tomatoes
- 4 cups vegetable broth (low sodium)
- 1 tablespoon olive oil
- 1 teaspoon oregano
- 1/2 teaspoon thyme
- Salt and pepper, to taste

Instructions:

1. Heat olive oil in a large pot over medium heat. Add the onion, carrots, celery, and garlic, and sauté for 5-7 minutes until softened.

2. Stir in the lentils, barley, oregano, thyme, salt, and pepper. Add the diced tomatoes and vegetable broth.

3. Bring the soup to a simmer and cook for 30-35 minutes until the lentils and barley are tender.

4. Adjust seasoning if needed. Serve hot.

Nutritional Value:
Calories 350 | Fat 7g | Saturated Fat 1g | Cholesterol 0mg | Sodium 470mg | Carbohydrate 60g | Fiber 15g | Added Sugar 0g | Protein 15g | Calcium 80mg | Potassium 700mg | Iron 4mg | Vitamin D 0mcg

White Bean and Turkey Sausage Soup

Prep Time: 10 minutes | **Cooking Time**: 30 minutes | **Total Time**: 40 minutes | **Serving**: 4 | **Cooking Difficulty**: Moderate

Ingredients:

- 1/2 pound turkey sausage, sliced
- 1 can (15 ounces) white beans, drained and rinsed
- 1 onion, diced
- 2 carrots, diced
- 2 celery stalks, diced
- 2 cloves garlic, minced
- 4 cups chicken broth (low sodium)
- 1/2 cup diced tomatoes
- 1 tablespoon olive oil
- 1 teaspoon oregano
- Salt and pepper, to taste

Instructions:

1. Heat olive oil in a large pot over medium heat. Add the sliced turkey sausage and cook for 5-7 minutes until browned. Remove from the pot and set aside.

2. In the same pot, add the onion, carrots, celery, and garlic, and sauté for 5 minutes until softened.

3. Stir in the oregano, salt, and pepper. Add the white beans, diced tomatoes, and chicken broth. Bring to a simmer and cook for 15 minutes.

4. Return the turkey sausage to the pot and cook for an additional 5 minutes.

5. Serve hot.

Nutritional Value:
Calories 350 | Fat 14g | Saturated Fat 3.5g | Cholesterol 50mg | Sodium 550mg | Carbohydrate 35g | Fiber 10g | Added Sugar 0g | Protein 25g | Calcium 80mg | Potassium 750mg | Iron 3.5mg | Vitamin D 0mcg

Kidney Bean and Beef Chili

Prep Time: 10 minutes | **Cooking Time:** 40 minutes | **Total Time:** 50 minutes | **Serving:** 4 | **Cooking Difficulty:** Moderate

Ingredients:

- 1 pound ground beef
- 1 can (15 ounces) kidney beans, drained and rinsed
- 1 onion, diced
- 1 bell pepper, diced
- 2 cloves garlic, minced
- 1 can (14 ounces) diced tomatoes
- 2 cups beef broth (low sodium)
- 1 tablespoon chili powder
- 1 teaspoon cumin
- 1/2 teaspoon smoked paprika
- Salt and pepper, to taste

Instructions:

1. Heat a large pot over medium heat. Add the ground beef and cook for 6-8 minutes until browned. Remove any excess fat.

2. Add the onion, bell pepper, and garlic to the pot, and sauté for 5 minutes until softened.

3. Stir in the chili powder, cumin, smoked paprika, salt, and pepper. Add the kidney beans, diced tomatoes, and beef broth.

4. Bring the chili to a simmer and cook for 30 minutes, stirring occasionally.

5. Serve hot.

Nutritional Value:
Calories 450 | Fat 20g | Saturated Fat 7g | Cholesterol 80mg | Sodium 600mg | Carbohydrate 35g | Fiber 12g | Added Sugar 0g | Protein 30g | Calcium 90mg | Potassium 800mg | Iron 5mg | Vitamin D 0mcg

Mung Bean and Tofu Hot Pot

Prep Time: 15 minutes | **Cooking Time:** 40 minutes | **Total Time:** 55 minutes | **Serving:** 4 | **Cooking Difficulty:** Moderate

Ingredients:

- 1 block (14 ounces) tofu, cubed
- 1/2 cup mung beans, soaked and rinsed
- 1 onion, diced
- 2 carrots, sliced
- 1 zucchini, sliced
- 2 cloves garlic, minced
- 4 cups vegetable broth (low sodium)
- 1 tablespoon soy sauce (low sodium)
- 1 tablespoon sesame oil
- 1 teaspoon ginger, minced
- Salt and pepper, to taste

Instructions:

1. Heat sesame oil in a large pot over medium heat. Add the cubed tofu and cook for 5-7 minutes until golden brown. Remove from the pot and set aside.

2. In the same pot, add the onion, carrots, zucchini, and garlic, and sauté for 5 minutes until softened.

3. Stir in the ginger, soy sauce, salt, and pepper. Add the mung beans and vegetable broth. Bring to a simmer and cook for 30 minutes until the mung beans are tender.

4. Return the tofu to the pot and cook for an additional 5 minutes.

5. Serve hot.

Nutritional Value:
Calories 350 | Fat 14g | Saturated Fat 2g | Cholesterol 0mg | Sodium 500mg | Carbohydrate 40g | Fiber 10g | Added Sugar 0g | Protein 20g | Calcium 250mg | Potassium 700mg | Iron 4mg | Vitamin D 0mcg

Casseroles

Turkey and Black Bean Enchilada Casserole

Prep Time: 15 minutes | **Cooking Time**: 30 minutes | **Total Time**: 45 minutes | **Serving**: 4 | **Cooking Difficulty**: Moderate

Ingredients:

- 1/2 pound ground turkey
- 1 can (15 ounces) black beans, drained and rinsed
- 1/2 cup enchilada sauce (store-bought or homemade)
- 8 small corn tortillas, cut into strips
- 1/2 cup shredded cheese (optional)
- 1/2 onion, diced
- 1/2 teaspoon cumin
- 1/2 teaspoon chili powder
- 1 tablespoon olive oil
- Salt and pepper, to taste

Instructions:

1. Preheat the oven to 375°F (190°C).
2. Heat olive oil in a skillet over medium heat. Add the diced onion and ground turkey, and cook for 6-8 minutes until the turkey is browned.
3. Stir in the cumin, chili powder, salt, and pepper. Add the black beans and cook for an additional 2-3 minutes.
4. In a baking dish, layer half the tortilla strips, followed by half the turkey and bean mixture, and half the enchilada sauce. Repeat with the remaining tortilla strips, turkey mixture, and sauce.
5. Top with shredded cheese if using.
6. Bake for 20-25 minutes until the casserole is bubbly and the cheese is melted. Serve hot.

Nutritional Value:

Calories 380 | Fat 15g | Saturated Fat 4g | Cholesterol 60mg | Sodium 500mg | Carbohydrate 40g | Fiber 10g | Added Sugar 0g | Protein 25g | Calcium 120mg | Potassium 750mg | Iron 3.5mg | Vitamin D 0mcg

Lentil and Sweet Potato Shepherd's Pie

Prep Time: 20 minutes | **Cooking Time**: 40 minutes | **Total Time**: 1 hour | **Serving**: 4 | **Cooking Difficulty**: Moderate

Ingredients:

- 1 cup cooked lentils
- 2 medium sweet potatoes, peeled and mashed
- 1 onion, diced
- 2 carrots, diced
- 1/2 cup green peas (fresh or frozen)
- 1 tablespoon olive oil
- 1 teaspoon thyme
- Salt and pepper, to taste

Instructions:

1. Preheat the oven to 375°F (190°C).

2. Heat olive oil in a skillet over medium heat. Add the onion and carrots, and sauté for 5-7 minutes until softened.

3. Stir in the cooked lentils, peas, thyme, salt, and pepper. Cook for an additional 3-4 minutes.

4. Transfer the lentil mixture to a baking dish. Spread the mashed sweet potatoes evenly over the top.

5. Bake for 20-25 minutes until the top is golden and the filling is heated through. Serve warm.

Nutritional Value:

Calories 350 | Fat 8g | Saturated Fat 1.5g | Cholesterol 0mg | Sodium 300mg | Carbohydrate 60g | Fiber 14g | Added Sugar 0g | Protein 10g | Calcium 90mg | Potassium 850mg | Iron 4mg | Vitamin D 0mcg

Chickpea and Chicken Bake

Prep Time: 15 minutes | **Cooking Time**: 35 minutes | **Total Time**: 50 minutes | **Serving**: 4 | **Cooking Difficulty**: Moderate

Ingredients:

- 2 chicken breasts, cubed
- 1 can (15 ounces) chickpeas, drained and rinsed
- 1/2 cup diced tomatoes
- 1/2 cup bell peppers, chopped
- 1/2 onion, diced
- 2 cloves garlic, minced
- 1 tablespoon olive oil
- 1 teaspoon paprika
- Salt and pepper, to taste

Instructions:

1. Preheat the oven to 375°F (190°C).

2. Heat olive oil in a skillet over medium heat. Add the onion, garlic, and bell peppers, and sauté for 5 minutes until softened.

3. Stir in the cubed chicken and cook for 6-8 minutes until browned.

4. Add the chickpeas, diced tomatoes, paprika, salt, and pepper. Stir to combine.

5. Transfer the mixture to a baking dish and bake for 25-30 minutes until the chicken is fully cooked and the sauce thickens.

6. Serve hot.

Nutritional Value:

Calories 400 | Fat 12g | Saturated Fat 2g | Cholesterol 65mg | Sodium 400mg | Carbohydrate 35g | Fiber 9g | Added Sugar 0g | Protein 35g | Calcium 60mg | Potassium 750mg | Iron 3mg | Vitamin D 0mcg

Quinoa Black Bean Mexican Casserole

Prep Time: 15 minutes | **Cooking Time**: 30 minutes | **Total Time**: 45 minutes | **Serving**: 4 | **Cooking Difficulty**: Easy

Ingredients:

- 1 cup cooked quinoa
- 1 can (15 ounces) black beans, drained and rinsed
- 1/2 cup corn kernels (fresh or frozen)
- 1/2 cup enchilada sauce
- 1/2 cup shredded cheese (optional)
- 1/2 teaspoon cumin
- 1/2 teaspoon chili powder
- 1 tablespoon olive oil
- Salt and pepper, to taste

Instructions:

1. Preheat the oven to 375°F (190°C).

2. In a large bowl, combine the cooked quinoa, black beans, corn, enchilada sauce, cumin, chili powder, salt, and pepper.

3. Transfer the mixture to a baking dish and top with shredded cheese if desired.

4. Bake for 25-30 minutes until the casserole is bubbly and the cheese is melted. Serve warm.

Nutritional Value:
Calories 350 | Fat 12g | Saturated Fat 4g | Cholesterol 15mg | Sodium 450mg | Carbohydrate 45g | Fiber 10g | Added Sugar 0g | Protein 15g | Calcium 120mg | Potassium 600mg | Iron 3mg | Vitamin D 0mcg

Tuna and White Bean Pasta Bake

Prep Time: 15 minutes | **Cooking Time**: 25 minutes | **Total Time**: 40 minutes | **Serving**: 4 | **Cooking Difficulty**: Moderate

Ingredients:

- 8 ounces whole wheat pasta

- 1 can (5 ounces) tuna in water, drained

- 1 can (15 ounces) white beans, drained and rinsed

- 1/2 cup diced tomatoes

- 1/2 cup shredded cheese (optional)

- 1/2 onion, diced

- 2 cloves garlic, minced

- 1 tablespoon olive oil

- 1 teaspoon oregano

- Salt and pepper, to taste

Instructions:

1. Preheat the oven to 375°F (190°C).

2. Cook the pasta according to package instructions. Drain and set aside.

3. Heat olive oil in a skillet over medium heat. Add the onion and garlic, and sauté for 5 minutes until softened.

4. Stir in the tuna, white beans, diced tomatoes, oregano, salt, and pepper. Cook for 3-4 minutes until heated through.

5. Mix the cooked pasta into the tuna and bean mixture.

6. Transfer the mixture to a baking dish and top with shredded cheese if desired.

7. Bake for 20-25 minutes until the casserole is bubbly and the cheese is melted. Serve hot.

Nutritional Value:
Calories 420 | Fat 12g | Saturated Fat 4g | Cholesterol 30mg | Sodium 500mg | Carbohydrate 55g | Fiber 12g | Added Sugar 0g | Protein 25g | Calcium 100mg | Potassium 700mg | Iron 4mg | Vitamin D 0mcg

Three Bean and Turkey Tamale Pie

Prep Time: 15 minutes | **Cooking Time**: 30 minutes | **Total Time**: 45 minutes | **Serving**: 4 | **Cooking Difficulty**: Moderate

Ingredients:

- 1/2 pound ground turkey

- 1/2 cup black beans, drained and rinsed

- 1/2 cup kidney beans, drained and rinsed

- 1/2 cup pinto beans, drained and rinsed

- 1/2 cup cornmeal

- 1/2 cup chicken broth (low sodium)

- 1/2 cup diced tomatoes

- 1/2 onion, diced

- 1 teaspoon cumin

- 1/2 teaspoon chili powder

- 1 tablespoon olive oil

- Salt and pepper, to taste

- 1/2 cup shredded cheese (optional)

Instructions:

1. Preheat the oven to 375°F (190°C).

2. Heat olive oil in a skillet over medium heat. Add diced onion and ground turkey. Cook for 6-8 minutes until the turkey is browned.

3. Stir in the cumin, chili powder, salt, pepper, black beans, kidney beans, pinto beans, and diced tomatoes. Cook for 2-3 minutes and set aside.

4. In a separate pot, bring the chicken broth to a boil and slowly whisk in the cornmeal. Cook for 2-3 minutes until thickened.

5. Pour the turkey and bean mixture into a baking dish and spread the cornmeal mixture on top.

6. Top with shredded cheese if desired.

7. Bake for 20-25 minutes until the top is golden and the pie is set. Serve warm.

Nutritional Value:
Calories 400 | Fat 14g | Saturated Fat 3.5g | Cholesterol 60mg | Sodium 500mg | Carbohydrate 45g | Fiber 12g | Added Sugar 0g | Protein 25g | Calcium 120mg | Potassium 800mg | Iron 4mg | Vitamin D 0mcg

Tempeh and Navy Bean Gratin

Prep Time: 15 minutes | **Cooking Time**: 25 minutes | **Total Time**: 40 minutes | **Serving**: 4 | **Cooking Difficulty**: Moderate

Ingredients:

- 1 block (8 ounces) tempeh, crumbled

- 1 cup cooked navy beans

- 1/2 cup breadcrumbs (whole wheat or gluten-free)

- 1/2 onion, diced

- 1 clove garlic, minced

- 1/4 cup grated Parmesan (optional)

- 1/4 teaspoon thyme

- 1 tablespoon olive oil

- Salt and pepper, to taste

Instructions:

1. Preheat the oven to 375°F (190°C).

2. Heat olive oil in a skillet over medium heat. Add the diced onion and garlic, and sauté for 5 minutes until softened.

3. Add the crumbled tempeh and cook for an additional 5 minutes until browned.

4. Stir in the cooked navy beans, thyme, salt, and pepper. Remove from heat.

5. Transfer the tempeh and bean mixture to a baking dish and top with breadcrumbs and Parmesan if using.

6. Bake for 20 minutes until the top is golden and crispy. Serve warm.

Nutritional Value:
Calories 360 | Fat 14g | Saturated Fat 3g | Cholesterol 5mg | Sodium 350mg | Carbohydrate 40g | Fiber 10g | Added Sugar 0g | Protein 20g | Calcium 120mg | Potassium 600mg | Iron 3mg | Vitamin D 0mcg

Edamame Rice Casserole

Prep Time: 10 minutes | **Cooking Time:** 30 minutes | **Total Time:** 40 minutes | **Serving:** 4 | **Cooking Difficulty:** Easy

Ingredients:

- 1 cup cooked brown rice
- 1/2 cup shelled edamame (fresh or frozen)
- 1/2 cup diced carrots
- 1/4 cup diced onions
- 1/2 cup shredded cheese (optional)
- 1 tablespoon soy sauce (low sodium)
- 1 tablespoon sesame oil
- 1 teaspoon garlic, minced
- Salt and pepper, to taste

Instructions:

1. Preheat the oven to 375°F (190°C).
2. Heat sesame oil in a skillet over medium heat. Add onions, carrots, and garlic. Sauté for 5 minutes until softened.
3. In a large bowl, combine the cooked brown rice, edamame, soy sauce, and the sautéed vegetables.
4. Transfer the mixture to a baking dish and top with shredded cheese if desired.
5. Bake for 20-25 minutes until heated through and the cheese is melted. Serve warm.

Nutritional Value:

Calories 320 | Fat 12g | Saturated Fat 3g | Cholesterol 10mg | Sodium 400mg | Carbohydrate 45g | Fiber 6g | Added Sugar 0g | Protein 12g | Calcium 80mg | Potassium 500mg | Iron 2.5mg | Vitamin D 0mcg

Lima Bean and Ham Layer Bake

Prep Time: 15 minutes | **Cooking Time:** 40 minutes | **Total Time:** 55 minutes | **Serving:** 4 | **Cooking Difficulty:** Moderate

Ingredients:

- 1 cup cooked lima beans
- 1/2 pound ham, diced
- 2 medium potatoes, thinly sliced
- 1/2 onion, diced
- 1/2 cup milk
- 1/2 cup shredded cheese (optional)
- 1 tablespoon olive oil
- Salt and pepper, to taste

Instructions:

1. Preheat the oven to 375°F (190°C).
2. Heat olive oil in a skillet over medium heat. Add diced onions and sauté for 5 minutes until softened.
3. In a baking dish, layer the sliced potatoes, lima beans, diced ham, and sautéed onions.
4. Pour the milk evenly over the layers and top with shredded cheese if desired.
5. Cover with foil and bake for 30 minutes. Remove the foil and bake for an additional 10 minutes until the top is golden and the potatoes are tender.
6. Serve warm.

Nutritional Value:

Calories 380 | Fat 15g | Saturated Fat 5g | Cholesterol 50mg | Sodium 600mg | Carbohydrate 45g | Fiber 7g | Added Sugar 0g | Protein 18g | Calcium 150mg | Potassium 850mg | Iron 3mg | Vitamin D 1mcg

Red Lentil Moussaka

Prep Time: 20 minutes | **Cooking Time:** 45 minutes | **Total Time:** 1 hour 5 minutes | **Serving:** 4 | **Cooking Difficulty:** Moderate

Ingredients:

- 1 cup red lentils, rinsed
- 1 eggplant, sliced
- 2 potatoes, sliced
- 1 onion, diced
- 2 cloves garlic, minced
- 1 can (14 ounces) diced tomatoes
- 1 tablespoon olive oil
- 1 teaspoon oregano
- Salt and pepper, to taste
- 1/2 cup béchamel sauce (optional)

Instructions:

1. Preheat the oven to 375°F (190°C).

2. Heat olive oil in a skillet over medium heat. Add the onion and garlic, and sauté for 5 minutes until softened.

3. Stir in the red lentils, diced tomatoes, oregano, salt, and pepper. Simmer for 15-20 minutes until the lentils are tender and the sauce thickens.

4. In a baking dish, layer the sliced potatoes, eggplant, and lentil mixture.

5. If using, pour the béchamel sauce over the top.

6. Bake for 30 minutes until the top is golden and the vegetables are tender. Serve warm.

Nutritional Value:

Calories 400 | Fat 12g | Saturated Fat 3g | Cholesterol 10mg | Sodium 450mg | Carbohydrate 60g | Fiber 14g | Added Sugar 0g | Protein 12g | Calcium 100mg | Potassium 850mg | Iron 4mg | Vitamin D 0mcg

Grain Bowls

Farro Black Bean Power Bowl

Prep Time: 10 minutes | **Cooking Time**: 20 minutes | **Total Time**: 30 minutes | **Serving**: 2 | **Cooking Difficulty**: Easy

Ingredients:

- 1/2 cup farro, rinsed
- 1/2 cup black beans, drained and rinsed
- 1/4 cup corn kernels (fresh or frozen)
- 1/2 avocado, sliced
- 1/4 cup cherry tomatoes, halved
- 1 tablespoon olive oil
- 1 tablespoon lime juice
- Salt and pepper, to taste
- Fresh cilantro, for garnish (optional)

Instructions:

1. Cook the farro according to package instructions. Drain and set aside.
2. In a serving bowl, combine the cooked farro, black beans, corn, avocado, and cherry tomatoes.
3. In a small bowl, whisk together olive oil, lime juice, salt, and pepper.
4. Drizzle the dressing over the bowl, toss gently, and garnish with fresh cilantro if desired. Serve immediately.

Nutritional Value:

Calories 400 | Fat 16g | Saturated Fat 2.5g | Cholesterol 0mg | Sodium 250mg | Carbohydrate 55g | Fiber 15g | Added Sugar 0g | Protein 12g | Calcium 80mg | Potassium 800mg | Iron 3mg | Vitamin D 0mcg

Barley Chickpea Buddha Bowl

Prep Time: 10 minutes | **Cooking Time**: 25 minutes | **Total Time**: 35 minutes | **Serving**: 2 | **Cooking Difficulty**: Easy

Ingredients:

- 1/2 cup pearl barley, rinsed
- 1/2 cup chickpeas, drained and rinsed
- 1/4 cup cucumber, diced
- 1/4 cup shredded carrots
- 1/2 avocado, sliced
- 1 tablespoon tahini
- 1 tablespoon lemon juice
- 1 tablespoon olive oil
- Salt and pepper, to taste
- Fresh parsley, for garnish (optional)

Instructions:

1. Cook the barley according to package instructions. Drain and set aside.
2. In a serving bowl, layer the cooked barley, chickpeas, cucumber, shredded carrots, and avocado.
3. In a small bowl, whisk together tahini, lemon juice, olive oil, salt, and pepper.
4. Drizzle the dressing over the bowl, toss lightly, and garnish with parsley if desired. Serve immediately.

Nutritional Value:

Calories 420 | Fat 18g | Saturated Fat 3g | Cholesterol 0mg | Sodium 200mg | Carbohydrate 55g | Fiber 12g |

Added Sugar 0g | Protein 14g | Calcium 100mg | Potassium 750mg | Iron 4mg | Vitamin D 0mcg

Quinoa Edamame Protein Bowl

Prep Time: 10 minutes | **Cooking Time**: 15 minutes | **Total Time**: 25 minutes | **Serving**: 2 | **Cooking Difficulty**: Easy

Ingredients:

- 1/2 cup quinoa, rinsed
- 1/2 cup shelled edamame
- 1/4 cup shredded cabbage
- 1/4 cup shredded carrots
- 1 tablespoon sesame oil
- 1 tablespoon soy sauce (low sodium)
- 1 tablespoon rice vinegar
- 1 teaspoon sesame seeds (optional)
- Salt and pepper, to taste

Instructions:

1. Cook the quinoa according to package instructions. Set aside.

2. Steam or boil the edamame until tender, then drain.

3. In a serving bowl, combine the quinoa, edamame, shredded cabbage, and shredded carrots.

4. In a small bowl, whisk together sesame oil, soy sauce, rice vinegar, salt, and pepper.

5. Drizzle the dressing over the bowl and toss lightly. Sprinkle with sesame seeds if desired. Serve immediately.

Nutritional Value:
Calories 360 | Fat 14g | Saturated Fat 2g | Cholesterol

0mg | Sodium 400mg | Carbohydrate 40g | Fiber 8g | Added Sugar 0g | Protein 15g | Calcium 80mg | Potassium 600mg | Iron 3mg | Vitamin D 0mcg

Brown Rice Lentil Energy Bowl

Prep Time: 10 minutes | **Cooking Time**: 25 minutes | **Total Time**: 35 minutes | **Serving**: 2 | **Cooking Difficulty**: Easy

Ingredients:

- 1/2 cup brown rice, cooked
- 1/2 cup cooked lentils
- 1/4 cup diced cucumber
- 1/4 cup cherry tomatoes, halved
- 1 tablespoon olive oil
- 1 tablespoon apple cider vinegar
- 1 teaspoon Dijon mustard
- Salt and pepper, to taste
- Fresh parsley, for garnish (optional)

Instructions:

1. In a serving bowl, layer the cooked brown rice, lentils, diced cucumber, and cherry tomatoes.

2. In a small bowl, whisk together olive oil, apple cider vinegar, Dijon mustard, salt, and pepper.

3. Drizzle the dressing over the bowl and toss lightly. Garnish with fresh parsley if desired. Serve immediately.

Nutritional Value:
Calories 380 | Fat 14g | Saturated Fat 2g | Cholesterol 0mg | Sodium 250mg | Carbohydrate 52g | Fiber 10g | Added Sugar 0g | Protein 12g | Calcium 70mg | Potassium 700mg | Iron 3.5mg | Vitamin D 0mcg

Bulgur White Bean Mediterranean Bowl

Prep Time: 10 minutes | **Cooking Time**: 15 minutes | **Total Time**: 25 minutes | **Serving**: 2 | **Cooking Difficulty**: Easy

Ingredients:

- 1/2 cup bulgur, rinsed
- 1/2 cup white beans, drained and rinsed
- 1/4 cup diced cucumber
- 1/4 cup cherry tomatoes, halved
- 1 tablespoon olive oil
- 1 tablespoon lemon juice
- 1 teaspoon oregano
- Salt and pepper, to taste
- Fresh mint, for garnish (optional)

Instructions:

1. Cook the bulgur according to package instructions. Drain and set aside.
2. In a serving bowl, layer the cooked bulgur, white beans, cucumber, and cherry tomatoes.
3. In a small bowl, whisk together olive oil, lemon juice, oregano, salt, and pepper.
4. Drizzle the dressing over the bowl and toss lightly. Garnish with fresh mint if desired. Serve immediately.

Nutritional Value:
Calories 370 | Fat 14g | Saturated Fat 2g | Cholesterol 0mg | Sodium 200mg | Carbohydrate 50g | Fiber 12g | Added Sugar 0g | Protein 12g | Calcium 80mg | Potassium 700mg | Iron 3.5mg | Vitamin D 0mcg

Millet Black-Eyed Pea Soul Bowl

Prep Time: 10 minutes | **Cooking Time**: 25 minutes | **Total Time**: 35 minutes | **Serving**: 2 | **Cooking Difficulty**: Easy

Ingredients:

- 1/2 cup millet, rinsed
- 1/2 cup cooked black-eyed peas
- 1/4 cup collard greens, chopped
- 1/4 cup shredded carrots
- 1 tablespoon olive oil
- 1 tablespoon apple cider vinegar
- 1 teaspoon hot sauce (optional)
- Salt and pepper, to taste
- Fresh parsley, for garnish (optional)

Instructions:

1. Cook the millet according to package instructions. Set aside.
2. In a skillet, sauté the collard greens with 1 teaspoon olive oil for 3-4 minutes until softened. Set aside.
3. In a serving bowl, layer the cooked millet, black-eyed peas, collard greens, and shredded carrots.
4. In a small bowl, whisk together olive oil, apple cider vinegar, hot sauce (if using), salt, and pepper.
5. Drizzle the dressing over the bowl, toss lightly, and garnish with fresh parsley if desired. Serve immediately.

Nutritional Value:
Calories 350 | Fat 14g | Saturated Fat 2g | Cholesterol 0mg | Sodium 250mg | Carbohydrate 45g | Fiber 10g | Added Sugar 0g | Protein 12g | Calcium 80mg | Potassium 700mg | Iron 3mg | Vitamin D 0mcg

Wild Rice Tempeh Harvest Bowl

Prep Time: 10 minutes | **Cooking Time**: 25 minutes | **Total Time**: 35 minutes | **Serving**: 2 | **Cooking Difficulty**: Moderate

Ingredients:

- 1/2 cup wild rice, rinsed
- 1 block (8 ounces) tempeh, cubed
- 1/4 cup roasted butternut squash
- 1/4 cup steamed broccoli
- 1 tablespoon olive oil
- 1 tablespoon balsamic vinegar
- 1 teaspoon maple syrup (optional)
- Salt and pepper, to taste

Instructions:

1. Cook the wild rice according to package instructions. Set aside.
2. In a skillet, heat 1 tablespoon olive oil and cook the tempeh cubes for 5-7 minutes until golden brown.
3. In a serving bowl, layer the cooked wild rice, tempeh, roasted butternut squash, and steamed broccoli.
4. In a small bowl, whisk together olive oil, balsamic vinegar, maple syrup (if using), salt, and pepper.
5. Drizzle the dressing over the bowl and toss lightly. Serve immediately.

Nutritional Value:
Calories 420 | Fat 18g | Saturated Fat 2.5g | Cholesterol 0mg | Sodium 250mg | Carbohydrate 50g | Fiber 10g | Added Sugar 0g | Protein 18g | Calcium 120mg | Potassium 700mg | Iron 4mg | Vitamin D 0mcg

Spelt Bean Burrito Bowl

Prep Time: 10 minutes | **Cooking Time**: 25 minutes | **Total Time**: 35 minutes | **Serving**: 2 | **Cooking Difficulty**: Easy

Ingredients:

- 1/2 cup cooked spelt
- 1/2 cup black beans, drained and rinsed
- 1/4 cup corn kernels (fresh or frozen)
- 1/4 cup diced tomatoes
- 1 tablespoon olive oil
- 1 tablespoon lime juice
- 1/2 teaspoon cumin
- Salt and pepper, to taste
- Fresh cilantro, for garnish (optional)

Instructions:

1. Cook the spelt according to package instructions. Set aside.
2. In a serving bowl, layer the cooked spelt, black beans, corn, and diced tomatoes.
3. In a small bowl, whisk together olive oil, lime juice, cumin, salt, and pepper.
4. Drizzle the dressing over the bowl, toss lightly, and garnish with fresh cilantro if desired. Serve immediately.

Nutritional Value:
Calories 380 | Fat 14g | Saturated Fat 2g | Cholesterol 0mg | Sodium 220mg | Carbohydrate 50g | Fiber 12g | Added Sugar 0g | Protein 15g | Calcium 80mg | Potassium 650mg | Iron 3.5mg | Vitamin D 0mcg

Amaranth Chickpea Breakfast Bowl

Prep Time: 10 minutes | **Cooking Time:** 20 minutes | **Total Time:** 30 minutes | **Serving:** 2 | **Cooking Difficulty:** Easy

Ingredients:

- 1/2 cup cooked amaranth
- 1/2 cup cooked chickpeas
- 1/4 cup diced cucumber
- 1/4 cup cherry tomatoes, halved
- 1 tablespoon olive oil
- 1 tablespoon lemon juice
- Salt and pepper, to taste
- Fresh mint, for garnish (optional)

Instructions:

1. Cook the amaranth according to package instructions. Set aside.
2. In a serving bowl, layer the cooked amaranth, chickpeas, diced cucumber, and cherry tomatoes.
3. In a small bowl, whisk together olive oil, lemon juice, salt, and pepper.
4. Drizzle the dressing over the bowl, toss lightly, and garnish with fresh mint if desired. Serve immediately.

Nutritional Value:

Calories 350 | Fat 12g | Saturated Fat 2g | Cholesterol 0mg | Sodium 220mg | Carbohydrate 50g | Fiber 10g | Added Sugar 0g | Protein 12g | Calcium 70mg | Potassium 600mg | Iron 3mg | Vitamin D 0mcg

Teff Lentil Ancient Grain Bowl

Prep Time: 10 minutes | **Cooking Time:** 25 minutes | **Total Time:** 35 minutes | **Serving:** 2 | **Cooking Difficulty:** Easy

Ingredients:

- 1/2 cup cooked teff
- 1/2 cup cooked lentils
- 1/4 cup shredded carrots
- 1/4 cup diced cucumbers
- 1 tablespoon olive oil
- 1 tablespoon apple cider vinegar
- 1/2 teaspoon Dijon mustard
- Salt and pepper, to taste
- Fresh parsley, for garnish (optional)

Instructions:

1. Cook the teff according to package instructions. Set aside.
2. In a serving bowl, layer the cooked teff, lentils, shredded carrots, and diced cucumbers.
3. In a small bowl, whisk together olive oil, apple cider vinegar, Dijon mustard, salt, and pepper.
4. Drizzle the dressing over the bowl, toss lightly, and garnish with fresh parsley if desired. Serve immediately.

Nutritional Value:

Calories 380 | Fat 14g | Saturated Fat 2g | Cholesterol 0mg | Sodium 230mg | Carbohydrate 55g | Fiber 12g | Added Sugar 0g | Protein 14g | Calcium 70mg | Potassium 700mg | Iron 3.5mg | Vitamin D 0mcg

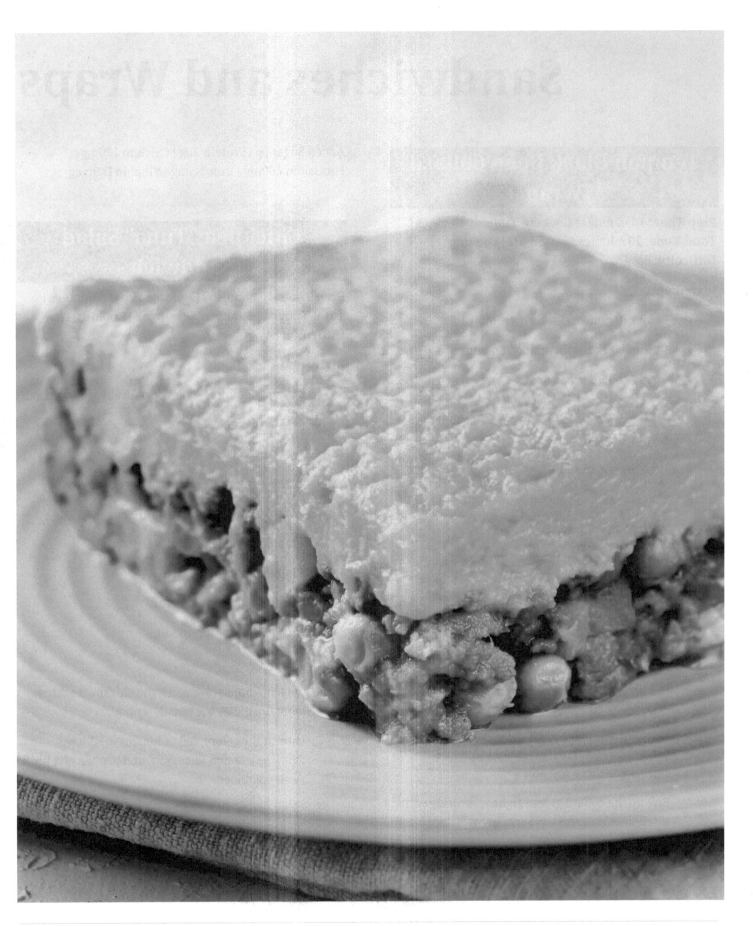

Sandwiches and Wraps

Tempeh Black Bean Collard Wrap

Prep Time: 10 minutes | **Cooking Time:** 10 minutes | **Total Time:** 20 minutes | **Serving:** 2 | **Cooking Difficulty:** Easy

Ingredients:

- 1 block (8 ounces) tempeh, crumbled
- 1/2 cup black beans, drained and rinsed
- 4 large collard green leaves
- 1/4 cup shredded carrots
- 1/4 cup diced tomatoes
- 1 tablespoon olive oil
- 1 tablespoon soy sauce (low sodium)
- 1 teaspoon cumin
- Salt and pepper, to taste

Instructions:

1. Heat olive oil in a skillet over medium heat. Add crumbled tempeh, cumin, salt, and pepper. Cook for 5-7 minutes until browned.

2. Stir in the black beans and soy sauce, and cook for another 2 minutes until heated through.

3. Place the tempeh and black bean mixture in the center of the collard leaves. Add shredded carrots and diced tomatoes.

4. Roll up the collard greens tightly, securing with toothpicks if necessary. Serve immediately.

Nutritional Value:
Calories 340 | Fat 14g | Saturated Fat 2.5g | Cholesterol 0mg | Sodium 400mg | Carbohydrate 35g | Fiber 12g | Added Sugar 0g | Protein 20g | Calcium 120mg | Potassium 600mg | Iron 3.5mg | Vitamin D 0mcg

Chickpea "Tuna" Salad Sandwich

Prep Time: 10 minutes | **Cooking Time:** 0 minutes | **Total Time:** 10 minutes | **Serving:** 2 | **Cooking Difficulty:** Easy

Ingredients:

- 1 can (15 ounces) chickpeas, drained and rinsed
- 1/4 cup diced celery
- 1/4 cup diced red onion
- 2 tablespoons vegan mayo or regular mayo
- 1 tablespoon Dijon mustard
- 1 tablespoon lemon juice
- Salt and pepper, to taste
- 4 slices whole grain bread
- Lettuce leaves (optional)

Instructions:

1. In a medium bowl, mash the chickpeas with a fork until they are mostly smooth.

2. Stir in the celery, red onion, mayo, Dijon mustard, lemon juice, salt, and pepper. Mix until well combined.

3. Spread the chickpea "tuna" mixture onto two slices of bread. Top with lettuce if desired, and place the remaining slices of bread on top to form sandwiches.

4. Serve immediately.

Nutritional Value:

Calories 350 | Fat 12g | Saturated Fat 1.5g | Cholesterol 5mg | Sodium 450mg | Carbohydrate 48g | Fiber 12g | Added Sugar 0g | Protein 12g | Calcium 80mg | Potassium 450mg | Iron 3mg | Vitamin D 0mcg

Lentil Walnut Burger

Prep Time: 15 minutes | **Cooking Time:** 10 minutes | **Total Time:** 25 minutes | **Serving:** 2 | **Cooking Difficulty:** Moderate

Ingredients:

- 1/2 cup cooked lentils
- 1/4 cup walnuts, finely chopped
- 1/4 cup breadcrumbs (whole wheat or gluten-free)
- 1 clove garlic, minced
- 1/2 teaspoon cumin
- 1 tablespoon olive oil (for cooking)
- Salt and pepper, to taste
- 2 whole grain burger buns
- Lettuce and tomato slices (optional, for serving)

Instructions:

1. In a large bowl, mash the cooked lentils with a fork until they are mostly smooth.
2. Stir in the chopped walnuts, breadcrumbs, garlic, cumin, salt, and pepper. Mix until well combined and form into two patties.
3. Heat olive oil in a skillet over medium heat. Cook the lentil patties for 4-5 minutes on each side until golden brown and heated through.
4. Serve the lentil burgers on whole grain buns with lettuce and tomato slices if desired.

Nutritional Value:

Calories 400 | Fat 18g | Saturated Fat 3g | Cholesterol

0mg | Sodium 400mg | Carbohydrate 45g | Fiber 12g | Added Sugar 0g | Protein 14g | Calcium 100mg | Potassium 600mg | Iron 3.5mg | Vitamin D 0mcg

Turkey Bean Sprout Wrap

Prep Time: 10 minutes | **Cooking Time:** 0 minutes | **Total Time:** 10 minutes | **Serving:** 2 | **Cooking Difficulty:** Easy

Ingredients:

- 4 slices deli turkey (low sodium)
- 1/2 cup bean sprouts
- 1/4 cup shredded carrots
- 2 whole grain tortillas
- 2 tablespoons hummus
- 1 tablespoon Dijon mustard
- Salt and pepper, to taste

Instructions:

1. Spread hummus evenly on each tortilla and drizzle with Dijon mustard.
2. Layer the turkey slices, bean sprouts, and shredded carrots on the tortillas.
3. Season with salt and pepper if desired, then roll up the tortillas tightly.
4. Slice in half and serve immediately.

Nutritional Value:

Calories 320 | Fat 10g | Saturated Fat 1.5g | Cholesterol 40mg | Sodium 600mg | Carbohydrate 35g | Fiber 8g | Added Sugar 0g | Protein 20g | Calcium 80mg | Potassium 400mg | Iron 2.5mg | Vitamin D 0mcg

White Bean and Tuna Pita

Prep Time: 10 minutes | **Cooking Time**: 0 minutes | **Total Time**: 10 minutes | **Serving**: 2 | **Cooking Difficulty**: Easy

Ingredients:

- 1 can (5 ounces) tuna in water, drained
- 1/2 cup white beans, drained and rinsed
- 1/4 cup diced cucumber
- 1/4 cup diced red onion
- 2 tablespoons olive oil
- 1 tablespoon lemon juice
- Salt and pepper, to taste
- 2 whole grain pitas

Instructions:

1. In a medium bowl, combine the tuna, white beans, cucumber, red onion, olive oil, lemon juice, salt, and pepper. Mix until well combined.
2. Cut the pitas in half and fill each half with the tuna and white bean mixture.
3. Serve immediately.

Nutritional Value:

Calories 350 | Fat 14g | Saturated Fat 2g | Cholesterol 30mg | Sodium 450mg | Carbohydrate 40g | Fiber 8g | Added Sugar 0g | Protein 22g | Calcium 80mg | Potassium 500mg | Iron 3mg | Vitamin D 0mcg

Edamame Hummus Veggie Wrap

Prep Time: 10 minutes | **Cooking Time**: 0 minutes | **Total Time**: 10 minutes | **Serving**: 2 | **Cooking Difficulty**: Easy

Ingredients:

- 1/2 cup edamame hummus (store-bought or homemade)
- 4 whole grain tortillas
- 1/2 cup shredded carrots
- 1/2 cucumber, sliced
- 1/4 cup alfalfa sprouts
- 1/4 avocado, sliced
- Salt and pepper, to taste

Instructions:

1. Spread the edamame hummus evenly over each tortilla.
2. Layer the shredded carrots, cucumber slices, alfalfa sprouts, and avocado in the center of the tortillas.
3. Season with salt and pepper.
4. Roll up the tortillas tightly, slice in half, and serve immediately.

Nutritional Value:

Calories 350 | Fat 14g | Saturated Fat 2g | Cholesterol 0mg | Sodium 350mg | Carbohydrate 45g | Fiber 10g | Added Sugar 0g | Protein 12g | Calcium 60mg | Potassium 600mg | Iron 3mg | Vitamin D 0mcg

Black Bean and Quinoa Burrito

Prep Time: 10 minutes | **Cooking Time**: 15 minutes | **Total Time**: 25 minutes | **Serving**: 2 | **Cooking Difficulty**: Easy

Ingredients:

- 1/2 cup cooked quinoa
- 1/2 cup black beans, drained and rinsed
- 1/4 cup corn kernels (fresh or frozen)
- 1/4 cup diced tomatoes
- 2 whole grain tortillas
- 1 tablespoon olive oil
- 1 teaspoon cumin
- Salt and pepper, to taste
- Fresh cilantro, for garnish (optional)

Instructions:

1. Heat olive oil in a skillet over medium heat. Add the black beans, corn, diced tomatoes, cumin, salt, and pepper. Cook for 5-7 minutes until heated through.
2. In a serving bowl, combine the cooked quinoa and black bean mixture.
3. Place the quinoa and black bean mixture in the center of each tortilla.
4. Roll up the tortillas tightly, slice in half, and garnish with fresh cilantro if desired. Serve immediately.

Nutritional Value:
Calories 400 | Fat 12g | Saturated Fat 2g | Cholesterol 0mg | Sodium 400mg | Carbohydrate 60g | Fiber 12g | Added Sugar 0g | Protein 14g | Calcium 80mg | Potassium 700mg | Iron 3.5mg | Vitamin D 0mcg

Navy Bean Chicken Salad Sandwich

Prep Time: 10 minutes | **Cooking Time**: 0 minutes | **Total Time**: 10 minutes | **Serving**: 2 | **Cooking Difficulty**: Easy

Ingredients:

- 1/2 cup cooked navy beans, mashed
- 1 cup cooked, shredded chicken breast
- 1/4 cup diced celery
- 2 tablespoons Greek yogurt
- 1 tablespoon Dijon mustard
- Salt and pepper, to taste
- 4 slices whole grain bread
- Lettuce leaves (optional)

Instructions:

1. In a medium bowl, combine the mashed navy beans, shredded chicken, celery, Greek yogurt, Dijon mustard, salt, and pepper. Mix until well combined.
2. Spread the chicken salad mixture evenly over two slices of bread.
3. Add lettuce if desired, and top with the remaining slices of bread to form sandwiches.
4. Serve immediately.

Nutritional Value:
Calories 350 | Fat 8g | Saturated Fat 1.5g | Cholesterol 50mg | Sodium 400mg | Carbohydrate 45g | Fiber 8g | Added Sugar 0g | Protein 28g | Calcium 60mg | Potassium 600mg | Iron 3mg | Vitamin D 0mcg

Red Lentil Falafel Wrap

Prep Time: 15 minutes | **Cooking Time:** 20 minutes | **Total Time:** 35 minutes | **Serving:** 2 | **Cooking Difficulty:** Moderate

Ingredients:

- 1 cup cooked red lentils
- 1/4 cup breadcrumbs (whole wheat or gluten-free)
- 1 clove garlic, minced
- 1/2 teaspoon cumin
- 1 tablespoon olive oil (for cooking)
- Salt and pepper, to taste
- 4 whole grain tortillas
- 1/4 cup shredded lettuce
- 1/4 cup diced tomatoes
- 2 tablespoons tahini (optional, for drizzle)

Instructions:

1. In a bowl, combine the cooked lentils, breadcrumbs, garlic, cumin, salt, and pepper. Form the mixture into small patties.

2. Heat olive oil in a skillet over medium heat. Cook the lentil patties for 4-5 minutes on each side until golden brown and crispy.

3. Place the lentil falafel patties in the center of the tortillas. Add shredded lettuce and diced tomatoes.

4. Drizzle with tahini if desired, roll up the tortillas, and serve immediately.

Nutritional Value:
Calories 380 | Fat 12g | Saturated Fat 2g | Cholesterol 0mg | Sodium 400mg | Carbohydrate 55g | Fiber 12g | Added Sugar 0g | Protein 14g | Calcium 80mg | Potassium 700mg | Iron 3.5mg | Vitamin D 0mcg

Split Pea Patty Sandwich

Prep Time: 15 minutes | **Cooking Time:** 15 minutes | **Total Time:** 30 minutes | **Serving:** 2 | **Cooking Difficulty:** Moderate

Ingredients:

- 1 cup cooked split peas
- 1/4 cup breadcrumbs (whole wheat or gluten-free)
- 1 clove garlic, minced
- 1 tablespoon olive oil (for cooking)
- 1/4 teaspoon thyme
- Salt and pepper, to taste
- 4 slices whole grain bread
- Lettuce and tomato slices (optional)

Instructions:

1. In a bowl, mash the cooked split peas with a fork. Stir in the breadcrumbs, garlic, thyme, salt, and pepper. Form the mixture into patties.

2. Heat olive oil in a skillet over medium heat. Cook the split pea patties for 4-5 minutes on each side until golden brown and heated through.

3. Serve the split pea patties on slices of whole grain bread with lettuce and tomato slices if desired. Serve immediately.

Nutritional Value:
Calories 360 | Fat 12g | Saturated Fat 2g | Cholesterol 0mg | Sodium 350mg | Carbohydrate 50g | Fiber 10g | Added Sugar 0g | Protein 14g | Calcium 80mg | Potassium 700mg | Iron 3.5mg | Vitamin D 0mcg

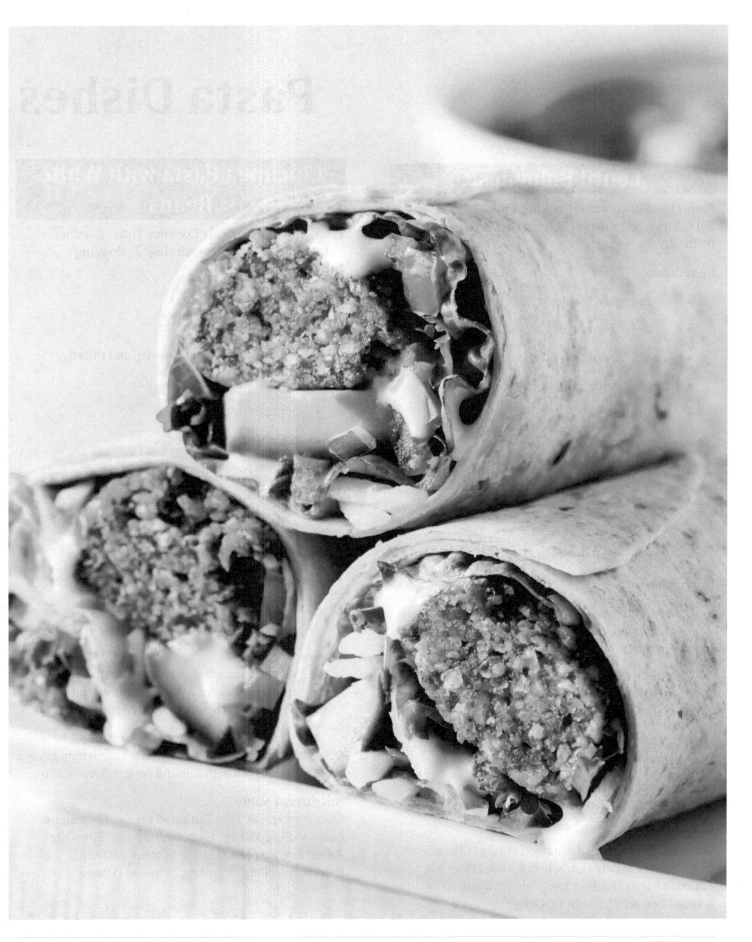

Pasta Dishes

Lentil Bolognese

Prep Time: 10 minutes | **Cooking Time:** 25 minutes | **Total Time:** 35 minutes | **Serving:** 4 | **Cooking Difficulty:** Easy

Ingredients:

- 1 cup cooked lentils
- 1 can (14 ounces) diced tomatoes
- 1 onion, diced
- 2 cloves garlic, minced
- 1 carrot, diced
- 1 tablespoon olive oil
- 1 teaspoon oregano
- 1/2 teaspoon thyme
- Salt and pepper, to taste
- 12 ounces whole wheat spaghetti

Instructions:

1. Heat olive oil in a skillet over medium heat. Add the onion, carrot, and garlic, and sauté for 5-7 minutes until softened.

2. Stir in the oregano, thyme, salt, and pepper. Add the diced tomatoes and cooked lentils. Simmer for 15 minutes until the sauce thickens.

3. Meanwhile, cook the spaghetti according to package instructions. Drain and set aside.

4. Serve the lentil Bolognese sauce over the cooked spaghetti. Serve warm.

Nutritional Value:
Calories 380 | Fat 10g | Saturated Fat 1.5g | Cholesterol 0mg | Sodium 350mg | Carbohydrate 60g | Fiber 12g | Added Sugar 0g | Protein 15g | Calcium 80mg | Potassium 800mg | Iron 4mg | Vitamin D 0mcg

Chickpea Pasta with White Beans

Prep Time: 10 minutes | **Cooking Time:** 15 minutes | **Total Time:** 25 minutes | **Serving:** 2 | **Cooking Difficulty:** Easy

Ingredients:

- 8 ounces chickpea pasta
- 1/2 cup white beans, drained and rinsed
- 1/2 cup cherry tomatoes, halved
- 1/4 cup fresh spinach
- 2 cloves garlic, minced
- 1 tablespoon olive oil
- 1 teaspoon lemon juice
- Salt and pepper, to taste

Instructions:

1. Cook the chickpea pasta according to package instructions. Drain and set aside.

2. In a skillet, heat olive oil over medium heat. Add garlic and sauté for 1-2 minutes until fragrant.

3. Add the white beans, cherry tomatoes, and spinach. Cook for 3-4 minutes until the spinach wilts and the beans are heated through.

4. Toss the cooked pasta with the sautéed vegetables and beans. Drizzle with lemon juice and season with salt and pepper. Serve warm.

Nutritional Value:
Calories 400 | Fat 12g | Saturated Fat 2g | Cholesterol 0mg | Sodium 350mg | Carbohydrate 60g | Fiber 10g | Added Sugar 0g | Protein 20g | Calcium 100mg | Potassium 700mg | Iron 4mg | Vitamin D 0mcg

Black Bean Pasta Primavera

Prep Time: 10 minutes | **Cooking Time:** 15 minutes | **Total Time:** 25 minutes | **Serving:** 2 | **Cooking Difficulty:** Easy

Ingredients:

- 8 ounces black bean pasta
- 1/2 cup broccoli florets
- 1/4 cup bell peppers, diced
- 1/4 cup zucchini, sliced
- 2 cloves garlic, minced
- 1 tablespoon olive oil
- 1 teaspoon Italian seasoning
- Salt and pepper, to taste
- 2 tablespoons grated Parmesan cheese (optional)

Instructions:

1. Cook the black bean pasta according to package instructions. Drain and set aside.
2. In a skillet, heat olive oil over medium heat. Add garlic, broccoli, bell peppers, and zucchini. Sauté for 5-7 minutes until the vegetables are tender.
3. Stir in Italian seasoning, salt, and pepper. Add the cooked pasta to the skillet and toss to combine.
4. Serve warm, garnished with Parmesan cheese if desired.

Nutritional Value:

Calories 380 | Fat 12g | Saturated Fat 2g | Cholesterol 0mg | Sodium 300mg | Carbohydrate 55g | Fiber 14g | Added Sugar 0g | Protein 22g | Calcium 90mg | Potassium 600mg | Iron 4mg | Vitamin D 0mcg

Edamame Noodle Stir-Fry

Prep Time: 10 minutes | **Cooking Time:** 10 minutes | **Total Time:** 20 minutes | **Serving:** 2 | **Cooking Difficulty:** Easy

Ingredients:

- 8 ounces soba noodles
- 1/2 cup shelled edamame
- 1/4 cup shredded carrots
- 1/4 cup bell peppers, sliced
- 1 tablespoon sesame oil
- 1 tablespoon soy sauce (low sodium)
- 1 teaspoon rice vinegar
- 1 clove garlic, minced
- Sesame seeds (optional, for garnish)

Instructions:

1. Cook soba noodles according to package instructions. Drain and set aside.
2. In a skillet, heat sesame oil over medium heat. Add garlic, carrots, and bell peppers, and sauté for 2-3 minutes until slightly softened.
3. Add the edamame, soy sauce, and rice vinegar. Cook for 3-4 minutes until the edamame is heated through.
4. Toss the cooked noodles with the stir-fried vegetables and serve immediately, garnished with sesame seeds if desired.

Nutritional Value:

Calories 370 | Fat 12g | Saturated Fat 2g | Cholesterol 0mg | Sodium 350mg | Carbohydrate 55g | Fiber 8g | Added Sugar 0g | Protein 18g | Calcium 80mg | Potassium 500mg | Iron 3mg | Vitamin D 0mcg

Red Lentil Penne with Turkey

Prep Time: 10 minutes | **Cooking Time**: 20 minutes | **Total Time**: 30 minutes | **Serving**: 4 | **Cooking Difficulty**: Moderate

Ingredients:

- 8 ounces red lentil penne
- 1/2 pound ground turkey
- 1/2 cup diced tomatoes
- 1/2 onion, diced
- 2 cloves garlic, minced
- 1 tablespoon olive oil
- 1 teaspoon oregano
- Salt and pepper, to taste
- Fresh basil, for garnish (optional)

Instructions:

1. Cook the red lentil penne according to package instructions. Drain and set aside.
2. In a skillet, heat olive oil over medium heat. Add the diced onion and garlic, and sauté for 5 minutes until softened.
3. Add the ground turkey and cook for 7-10 minutes until browned. Stir in the diced tomatoes, oregano, salt, and pepper. Simmer for 5 minutes.
4. Toss the cooked penne with the turkey sauce. Garnish with fresh basil if desired. Serve warm.

Nutritional Value:
Calories 400 | Fat 12g | Saturated Fat 2.5g | Cholesterol 55mg | Sodium 400mg | Carbohydrate 50g | Fiber 10g | Added Sugar 0g | Protein 30g | Calcium 100mg | Potassium 700mg | Iron 3mg | Vitamin D 0mcg

Three Bean Pasta Salad

Prep Time: 10 minutes | **Cooking Time**: 10 minutes | **Total Time**: 20 minutes | **Serving**: 4 | **Cooking Difficulty**: Easy

Ingredients:

- 8 ounces whole wheat pasta
- 1/2 cup black beans, drained and rinsed
- 1/2 cup kidney beans, drained and rinsed
- 1/2 cup chickpeas, drained and rinsed
- 1/4 cup cherry tomatoes, halved
- 1/4 cup diced cucumber
- 2 tablespoons olive oil
- 2 tablespoons lemon juice
- 1 teaspoon Dijon mustard
- Salt and pepper, to taste

Instructions:

1. Cook the pasta according to package instructions. Drain and set aside.
2. In a large bowl, combine the black beans, kidney beans, chickpeas, cherry tomatoes, and cucumber.
3. In a small bowl, whisk together olive oil, lemon juice, Dijon mustard, salt, and pepper.
4. Toss the cooked pasta with the bean mixture and drizzle with the dressing. Serve chilled or at room temperature.

Nutritional Value:
Calories 380 | Fat 12g | Saturated Fat 2g | Cholesterol 0mg | Sodium 250mg | Carbohydrate 60g | Fiber 12g | Added Sugar 0g | Protein 15g | Calcium 80mg | Potassium 700mg | Iron 3.5mg | Vitamin D 0mcg

Tempeh Marinara with Legume Pasta

Prep Time: 10 minutes | **Cooking Time**: 20 minutes | **Total Time**: 30 minutes | **Serving**: 2 | **Cooking Difficulty**: Easy

Ingredients:

- 8 ounces legume-based pasta (e.g., chickpea or lentil pasta)
- 1 block (8 ounces) tempeh, crumbled
- 1/2 cup marinara sauce (store-bought or homemade)
- 1/2 onion, diced
- 2 cloves garlic, minced
- 1 tablespoon olive oil
- 1 teaspoon oregano
- Salt and pepper, to taste
- Fresh basil, for garnish (optional)

Instructions:

1. Cook the legume pasta according to package instructions. Drain and set aside.
2. Heat olive oil in a skillet over medium heat. Add diced onion and garlic, and sauté for 5 minutes until softened.
3. Add the crumbled tempeh, oregano, salt, and pepper. Cook for 5-7 minutes until the tempeh is browned.
4. Stir in the marinara sauce and cook for an additional 5 minutes until heated through.
5. Toss the cooked pasta with the tempeh marinara and serve warm, garnished with fresh basil if desired.

Nutritional Value:
Calories 420 | Fat 14g | Saturated Fat 2g | Cholesterol 0mg | Sodium 450mg | Carbohydrate 50g | Fiber 14g | Added Sugar 0g | Protein 25g | Calcium 120mg | Potassium 750mg | Iron 4mg | Vitamin D 0mcg

Navy Bean Mac and Cheese

Prep Time: 10 minutes | **Cooking Time**: 20 minutes | **Total Time**: 30 minutes | **Serving**: 4 | **Cooking Difficulty**: Moderate

Ingredients:

- 8 ounces whole wheat elbow pasta
- 1 cup cooked navy beans
- 1/2 cup shredded cheese (cheddar or vegan alternative)
- 1/2 cup milk (or dairy-free milk)
- 2 tablespoons nutritional yeast (optional)
- 1 tablespoon olive oil
- 1 tablespoon flour (all-purpose or gluten-free)
- Salt and pepper, to taste

Instructions:

1. Cook the pasta according to package instructions. Drain and set aside.
2. In a saucepan, heat olive oil over medium heat. Stir in the flour to make a roux and cook for 1-2 minutes.
3. Slowly whisk in the milk and cook until the mixture thickens, about 3-4 minutes.
4. Stir in the shredded cheese, nutritional yeast (if using), navy beans, salt, and pepper. Cook until the cheese is fully melted.
5. Toss the cooked pasta with the cheese and bean sauce, and serve warm.

Nutritional Value:
Calories 400 | Fat 14g | Saturated Fat 4g | Cholesterol 20mg | Sodium 450mg | Carbohydrate 55g | Fiber 10g | Added Sugar 0g | Protein 18g | Calcium 200mg | Potassium 600mg | Iron 3mg | Vitamin D 1mcg

Mung Bean Glass Noodle Bowl

Prep Time: 10 minutes | **Cooking Time**: 10 minutes | **Total Time**: 20 minutes | **Serving**: 2 | **Cooking Difficulty**: Easy

Ingredients:

- 4 ounces glass noodles
- 1/2 cup cooked mung beans
- 1/4 cup shredded carrots
- 1/4 cup sliced bell peppers
- 1 tablespoon soy sauce (low sodium)
- 1 tablespoon sesame oil
- 1 teaspoon rice vinegar
- 1 clove garlic, minced
- Sesame seeds (optional, for garnish)

Instructions:

1. Cook the glass noodles according to package instructions. Drain and set aside.
2. In a bowl, combine the mung beans, shredded carrots, and bell peppers.
3. In a small bowl, whisk together soy sauce, sesame oil, rice vinegar, and minced garlic.
4. Toss the noodles with the vegetables and mung beans, then drizzle with the dressing.
5. Garnish with sesame seeds if desired and serve warm or at room temperature.

Nutritional Value:
Calories 320 | Fat 12g | Saturated Fat 2g | Cholesterol 0mg | Sodium 400mg | Carbohydrate 45g | Fiber 8g | Added Sugar 0g | Protein 12g | Calcium 60mg | Potassium 450mg | Iron 2.5mg | Vitamin D 0mcg

Lima Bean Pasta Alfredo

Prep Time: 10 minutes | **Cooking Time**: 20 minutes | **Total Time**: 30 minutes | **Serving**: 2 | **Cooking Difficulty**: Moderate

Ingredients:

- 8 ounces whole wheat fettuccine
- 1/2 cup cooked lima beans
- 1/2 cup heavy cream (or dairy-free alternative)
- 1/4 cup grated Parmesan cheese (or vegan alternative)
- 1 tablespoon olive oil
- 2 cloves garlic, minced
- Salt and pepper, to taste
- Fresh parsley, for garnish (optional)

Instructions:

1. Cook the fettuccine according to package instructions. Drain and set aside.
2. In a skillet, heat olive oil over medium heat. Add the minced garlic and sauté for 1-2 minutes until fragrant.
3. Stir in the heavy cream and bring to a simmer. Add the grated Parmesan cheese and stir until melted and smooth.
4. Stir in the cooked lima beans, season with salt and pepper, and cook for 2-3 minutes.
5. Toss the cooked fettuccine with the Alfredo sauce and serve warm, garnished with fresh parsley if desired.

Nutritional Value:
Calories 420 | Fat 18g | Saturated Fat 8g | Cholesterol 40mg | Sodium 400mg | Carbohydrate 55g | Fiber 10g | Added Sugar 0g | Protein 15g | Calcium 150mg | Potassium 550mg | Iron 3mg | Vitamin D 0mcg

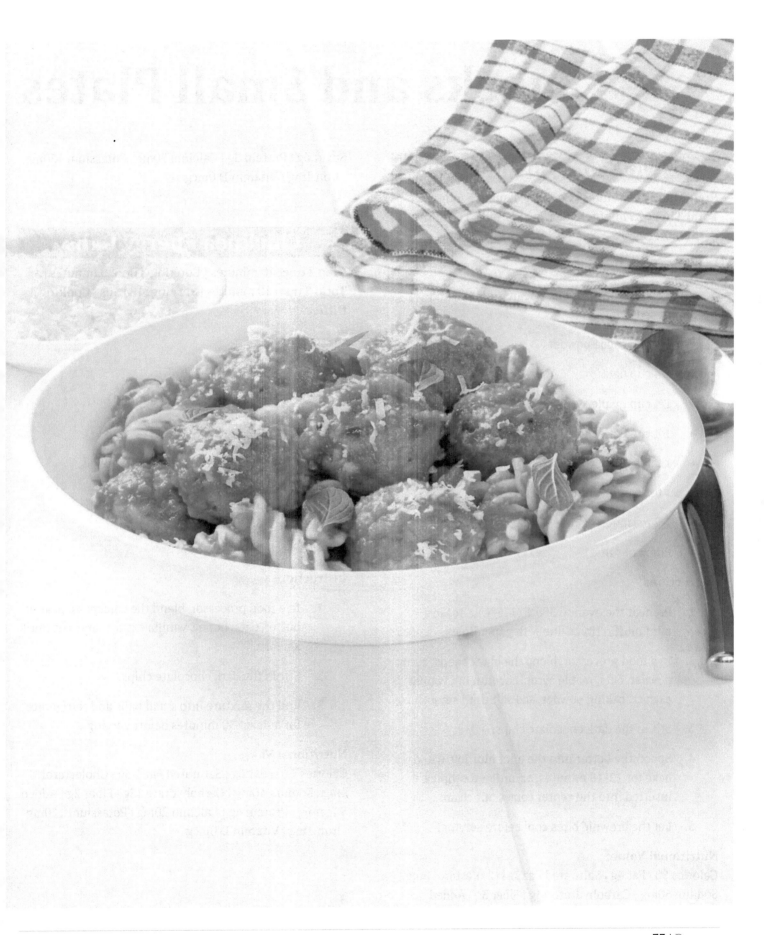

Snacks and Small Plates

Black Bean Brownie Bites

Prep Time: 10 minutes | **Cooking Time:** 15 minutes | **Total Time:** 25 minutes | **Serving:** 12 bites | **Cooking Difficulty:** Easy

Ingredients:

- 1 can (15 ounces) black beans, drained and rinsed
- 1/4 cup cocoa powder
- 1/4 cup oats
- 1/4 cup maple syrup
- 1/4 cup dark chocolate chips
- 1 tablespoon coconut oil
- 1 teaspoon vanilla extract
- 1/2 teaspoon baking powder
- Pinch of salt

Instructions:

1. Preheat the oven to 350°F (175°C). Grease a mini muffin tin or line with paper liners.
2. In a food processor, blend the black beans, cocoa powder, oats, maple syrup, coconut oil, vanilla extract, baking powder, and salt until smooth.
3. Stir in the dark chocolate chips.
4. Spoon the batter into the mini muffin tin and bake for 12-15 minutes, or until a toothpick inserted into the center comes out clean.
5. Let the brownie bites cool before serving.

Nutritional Value:
Calories 90 | Fat 4g | Saturated Fat 2g | Cholesterol 0mg | Sodium 60mg | Carbohydrate 14g | Fiber 3g | Added Sugar 6g | Protein 3g | Calcium 20mg | Potassium 150mg | Iron 1mg | Vitamin D 0mcg

Chickpea Energy Balls

Prep Time: 10 minutes | **Cooking Time:** 0 minutes | **Total Time:** 10 minutes | **Serving:** 12 balls | **Cooking Difficulty:** Easy

Ingredients:

- 1 cup cooked chickpeas
- 1/4 cup peanut butter or almond butter
- 1/4 cup rolled oats
- 2 tablespoons honey or maple syrup
- 1/4 cup dark chocolate chips
- 1/2 teaspoon vanilla extract
- Pinch of salt

Instructions:

1. In a food processor, blend the chickpeas, peanut butter, oats, honey, vanilla extract, and salt until smooth.
2. Stir in the dark chocolate chips.
3. Roll the mixture into small balls and refrigerate for at least 30 minutes before serving.

Nutritional Value:
Calories 120 | Fat 6g | Saturated Fat 1.5g | Cholesterol 0mg | Sodium 40mg | Carbohydrate 15g | Fiber 2g | Added Sugar 6g | Protein 4g | Calcium 20mg | Potassium 120mg | Iron 1mg | Vitamin D 0mcg

Lentil Crackers

Prep Time: 10 minutes | **Cooking Time:** 20 minutes | **Total Time:** 30 minutes | **Serving:** 20 crackers | **Cooking Difficulty:** Moderate

Ingredients:

- 1 cup cooked lentils
- 1/2 cup chickpea flour
- 1 tablespoon olive oil
- 1 teaspoon garlic powder
- 1/2 teaspoon salt
- 1/4 teaspoon black pepper
- 1/2 teaspoon dried oregano (optional)

Instructions:

1. Preheat the oven to 350°F (175°C) and line a baking sheet with parchment paper.
2. In a food processor, blend the lentils, chickpea flour, olive oil, garlic powder, salt, pepper, and oregano (if using) until a dough forms.
3. Roll the dough between two sheets of parchment paper to about 1/8-inch thickness. Cut into squares or shapes using a knife or cookie cutter.
4. Place the crackers on the prepared baking sheet and bake for 15-20 minutes, or until crisp and golden.
5. Let the crackers cool before serving.

Nutritional Value:
Calories 50 | Fat 2g | Saturated Fat 0g | Cholesterol 0mg | Sodium 80mg | Carbohydrate 8g | Fiber 2g | Added Sugar 0g | Protein 2g | Calcium 10mg | Potassium 100mg | Iron 0.5mg | Vitamin D 0mcg

Edamame Hummus

Prep Time: 10 minutes | **Cooking Time:** 0 minutes | **Total Time:** 10 minutes | **Serving:** 6 | **Cooking Difficulty:** Easy

Ingredients:

- 1 cup shelled edamame (cooked)
- 1/4 cup tahini
- 1/4 cup olive oil
- 2 tablespoons lemon juice
- 1 clove garlic, minced
- 1/2 teaspoon salt
- 1/4 teaspoon ground cumin
- 1-2 tablespoons water (as needed)

Instructions:

1. In a food processor, blend the edamame, tahini, olive oil, lemon juice, garlic, salt, and cumin until smooth.
2. Add water, 1 tablespoon at a time, until the hummus reaches your desired consistency.
3. Serve with veggies, pita, or crackers.

Nutritional Value:
Calories 150 | Fat 12g | Saturated Fat 1.5g | Cholesterol 0mg | Sodium 200mg | Carbohydrate 8g | Fiber 3g | Added Sugar 0g | Protein 5g | Calcium 40mg | Potassium 150mg | Iron 1mg | Vitamin D 0mcg

Three Bean Dip

Prep Time: 10 minutes | **Cooking Time:** 0 minutes | **Total Time:** 10 minutes | **Serving:** 4 | **Cooking Difficulty:** Easy

Ingredients:

- 1/2 cup black beans, drained and rinsed
- 1/2 cup kidney beans, drained and rinsed
- 1/2 cup pinto beans, drained and rinsed
- 1/4 cup salsa
- 1/4 cup Greek yogurt or vegan yogurt
- 1 teaspoon lime juice
- 1/2 teaspoon cumin
- Salt and pepper, to taste

Instructions:

1. In a food processor, blend the black beans, kidney beans, pinto beans, salsa, yogurt, lime juice, cumin, salt, and pepper until smooth.

2. Serve with tortilla chips, veggies, or as a spread for sandwiches.

Nutritional Value:

Calories 120 | Fat 3g | Saturated Fat 1g | Cholesterol 5mg | Sodium 240mg | Carbohydrate 20g | Fiber 6g | Added Sugar 0g | Protein 6g | Calcium 60mg | Potassium 250mg | Iron 2mg | Vitamin D 0mcg

Roasted Lupini Beans

Prep Time: 5 minutes | **Cooking Time:** 30 minutes | **Total Time:** 35 minutes | **Serving:** 4 | **Cooking Difficulty:** Easy

Ingredients:

- 1 cup lupini beans, cooked and drained
- 1 tablespoon olive oil
- 1/2 teaspoon smoked paprika
- 1/2 teaspoon garlic powder
- Salt and pepper, to taste

Instructions:

1. Preheat the oven to 375°F (190°C).

2. In a bowl, toss the lupini beans with olive oil, smoked paprika, garlic powder, salt, and pepper.

3. Spread the beans evenly on a baking sheet lined with parchment paper.

4. Roast for 25-30 minutes, stirring occasionally, until the beans are golden and crispy.

5. Allow to cool slightly before serving.

Nutritional Value:

Calories 120 | Fat 6g | Saturated Fat 1g | Cholesterol 0mg | Sodium 200mg | Carbohydrate 10g | Fiber 4g | Added Sugar 0g | Protein 10g | Calcium 30mg | Potassium 100mg | Iron 1.5mg | Vitamin D 0mcg

Tempeh "Wings"

Prep Time: 10 minutes | **Cooking Time:** 20 minutes | **Total Time:** 30 minutes | **Serving:** 4 | **Cooking Difficulty:** Moderate

Ingredients:

- 1 block (8 ounces) tempeh, cut into strips
- 1/4 cup soy sauce (low sodium)
- 2 tablespoons maple syrup
- 1 tablespoon olive oil
- 1 teaspoon smoked paprika
- 1/2 teaspoon garlic powder
- 1/2 teaspoon chili powder
- 1 tablespoon hot sauce (optional, for extra heat)

Instructions:

1. Preheat the oven to 375°F (190°C) and line a baking sheet with parchment paper.

2. In a bowl, whisk together soy sauce, maple syrup, olive oil, smoked paprika, garlic powder, chili powder, and hot sauce (if using).

3. Toss the tempeh strips in the marinade until well coated.

4. Spread the tempeh strips evenly on the prepared baking sheet.

5. Bake for 20 minutes, flipping halfway through, until the tempeh is crispy and golden.

6. Serve with your favorite dipping sauce.

Nutritional Value:

Calories 220 | Fat 11g | Saturated Fat 1.5g | Cholesterol 0mg | Sodium 350mg | Carbohydrate 18g | Fiber 3g | Added Sugar 6g | Protein 15g | Calcium 50mg | Potassium 200mg | Iron 3mg | Vitamin D 0mcg

Quinoa Protein Bars

Prep Time: 10 minutes | **Cooking Time**: 0 minutes | **Total Time**: 10 minutes (plus chilling time) | **Serving**: 8 bars | **Cooking Difficulty**: Easy

Ingredients:

- 1/2 cup cooked quinoa

- 1/2 cup rolled oats

- 1/4 cup almond butter or peanut butter

- 1/4 cup honey or maple syrup

- 1/4 cup protein powder (optional)

- 1/4 cup dark chocolate chips

- 1/2 teaspoon vanilla extract

- Pinch of salt

Instructions:

1. In a large bowl, mix the cooked quinoa, oats, almond butter, honey, protein powder (if using), vanilla extract, and salt until well combined.

2. Stir in the dark chocolate chips.

3. Press the mixture firmly into an 8x8-inch baking dish lined with parchment paper.

4. Refrigerate for at least 1 hour to firm up.

5. Slice into bars and store in the refrigerator.

Nutritional Value:

Calories 220 | Fat 10g | Saturated Fat 2.5g | Cholesterol 0mg | Sodium 60mg | Carbohydrate 26g | Fiber 4g | Added Sugar 10g | Protein 8g | Calcium 40mg | Potassium 200mg | Iron 2mg | Vitamin D 0mcg

Black-Eyed Pea Fritters

Prep Time: 10 minutes | **Cooking Time**: 10 minutes | **Total Time**: 20 minutes | **Serving**: 4 | **Cooking Difficulty**: Moderate

Ingredients:

- 1 cup cooked black-eyed peas

- 1/4 cup chickpea flour

- 1 clove garlic, minced

- 1/4 teaspoon cumin

- 1/4 teaspoon paprika

- 1 tablespoon olive oil (for frying)

- Salt and pepper, to taste

Instructions:

1. In a large bowl, mash the black-eyed peas with a fork until mostly smooth.

2. Stir in the chickpea flour, garlic, cumin, paprika, salt, and pepper until a dough forms.

3. Form the mixture into small patties or balls.

4. Heat olive oil in a skillet over medium heat. Fry the fritters for 3-4 minutes on each side until golden and crispy.

5. Serve warm with your favorite dipping sauce.

Nutritional Value:
Calories 160 | Fat 7g | Saturated Fat 1g | Cholesterol 0mg | Sodium 150mg | Carbohydrate 20g | Fiber 5g | Added Sugar 0g | Protein 6g | Calcium 40mg | Potassium 250mg | Iron 1.5mg | Vitamin D 0mcg

Spiced Roasted Chickpeas

Prep Time: 5 minutes | **Cooking Time**: 25 minutes | **Total Time**: 30 minutes | **Serving**: 4 | **Cooking Difficulty**: Easy

Ingredients:

- 1 can (15 ounces) chickpeas, drained and rinsed

- 1 tablespoon olive oil

- 1/2 teaspoon smoked paprika

- 1/2 teaspoon garlic powder

- 1/2 teaspoon cumin

- Salt and pepper, to taste

Instructions:

1. Preheat the oven to 400°F (200°C) and line a baking sheet with parchment paper.

2. Pat the chickpeas dry with a paper towel.

3. Toss the chickpeas with olive oil, smoked paprika, garlic powder, cumin, salt, and pepper until evenly coated.

4. Spread the chickpeas on the prepared baking sheet in a single layer.

5. Roast for 20-25 minutes, shaking the pan halfway through, until the chickpeas are golden and crispy.

6. Let cool slightly before serving.

Nutritional Value:
Calories 150 | Fat 7g | Saturated Fat 1g | Cholesterol 0mg | Sodium 180mg | Carbohydrate 20g | Fiber 6g | Added Sugar 0g | Protein 5g | Calcium 40mg | Potassium 240mg | Iron 1.5mg | Vitamin D 0mcg

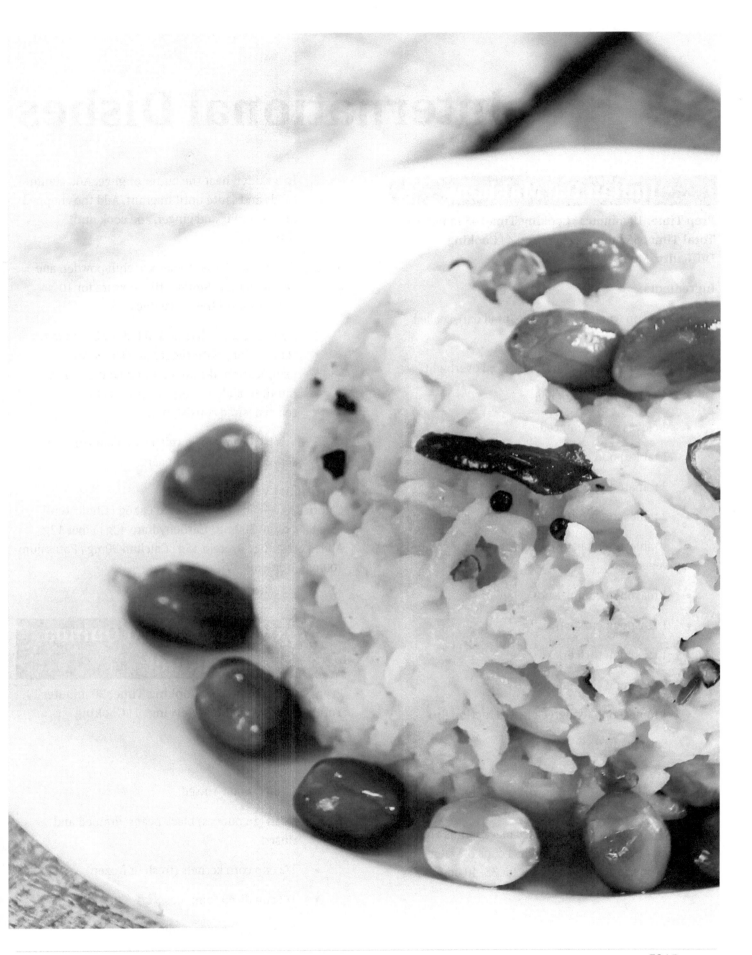

International Dishes

Indian Dal Makhani

Prep Time: 10 minutes | **Cooking Time:** 45 minutes | **Total Time:** 55 minutes | **Serving:** 4 | **Cooking Difficulty:** Moderate

Ingredients:

- 1/2 cup whole black lentils (urad dal), soaked overnight
- 1/4 cup red kidney beans, soaked overnight
- 1 onion, finely chopped
- 2 cloves garlic, minced
- 1 tablespoon ginger, minced
- 2 tomatoes, pureed
- 2 tablespoons butter or ghee (or vegan butter)
- 1 tablespoon heavy cream (or coconut cream for vegan)
- 1 teaspoon cumin seeds
- 1 teaspoon garam masala
- 1 teaspoon turmeric
- 1 teaspoon chili powder
- 1 tablespoon fenugreek leaves (optional)
- Salt, to taste
- Fresh cilantro for garnish

Instructions:

1. Drain and rinse the soaked black lentils and kidney beans. Boil them in 4 cups of water with turmeric and salt. Simmer for 35-40 minutes until tender.

2. In a skillet, heat the butter or ghee. Add cumin seeds and sauté until fragrant. Add the chopped onion, garlic, and ginger, and cook until softened.

3. Stir in the pureed tomatoes, chili powder, and garam masala. Simmer the mixture for 10 minutes until the sauce thickens.

4. Add the cooked lentils and kidney beans to the skillet, along with the fenugreek leaves (if using). Stir and simmer for an additional 10 minutes, adding more water if necessary to reach desired consistency.

5. Stir in the cream, garnish with cilantro, and serve hot with rice or naan.

Nutritional Value:

Calories 320 | Fat 14g | Saturated Fat 6g | Cholesterol 25mg | Sodium 300mg | Carbohydrate 40g | Fiber 12g | Added Sugar 0g | Protein 15g | Calcium 90mg | Potassium 700mg | Iron 4mg | Vitamin D 0mcg

Mexican Bean and Quinoa Skillet

Prep Time: 10 minutes | **Cooking Time:** 20 minutes | **Total Time:** 30 minutes | **Serving:** 4 | **Cooking Difficulty:** Easy

Ingredients:

- 1 cup quinoa, rinsed
- 1 can (15 ounces) black beans, drained and rinsed
- 1/2 cup corn kernels (fresh or frozen)
- 1/2 cup diced tomatoes
- 1/4 cup bell peppers, diced

- 1 teaspoon cumin
- 1 teaspoon chili powder
- 1 tablespoon olive oil
- Salt and pepper, to taste
- Fresh cilantro, for garnish (optional)
- Lime wedges, for serving

Instructions:

1. In a large skillet, heat olive oil over medium heat. Add the quinoa and toast for 2-3 minutes.

2. Add 2 cups of water, cumin, chili powder, salt, and pepper. Bring to a boil, then reduce heat and simmer for 15 minutes until the quinoa is cooked.

3. Stir in the black beans, corn, diced tomatoes, and bell peppers. Cook for 3-5 minutes until heated through.

4. Garnish with fresh cilantro and serve with lime wedges.

Nutritional Value:

Calories 350 | Fat 10g | Saturated Fat 1.5g | Cholesterol 0mg | Sodium 400mg | Carbohydrate 52g | Fiber 12g | Added Sugar 0g | Protein 12g | Calcium 80mg | Potassium 700mg | Iron 4mg | Vitamin D 0mcg

Ethiopian Red Lentil Stew (Misir Wot)

Prep Time: 10 minutes | **Cooking Time:** 30 minutes | **Total Time:** 40 minutes | **Serving:** 4 | **Cooking Difficulty:** Moderate

Ingredients:

- 1 cup red lentils, rinsed
- 1 onion, finely chopped
- 2 cloves garlic, minced
- 1 tablespoon ginger, minced
- 1 tablespoon berbere spice (or to taste)
- 2 tablespoons olive oil
- 2 tomatoes, pureed
- 1/2 teaspoon cumin
- 4 cups vegetable broth or water
- Salt, to taste
- Injera or rice, for serving

Instructions:

1. In a large pot, heat olive oil over medium heat. Add the chopped onion, garlic, and ginger, and sauté for 5 minutes until softened.

2. Stir in the berbere spice and cumin, and cook for another 1-2 minutes until fragrant.

3. Add the pureed tomatoes and cook for 5 minutes until the sauce thickens.

4. Add the rinsed red lentils and vegetable broth. Bring to a simmer and cook for 20-25 minutes, stirring occasionally, until the lentils are tender and the stew thickens.

5. Season with salt and serve hot with injera or rice.

Nutritional Value:

Calories 290 | Fat 10g | Saturated Fat 1.5g | Cholesterol 0mg | Sodium 500mg | Carbohydrate 40g | Fiber 12g | Added Sugar 0g | Protein 14g | Calcium 60mg | Potassium 600mg | Iron 3.5mg | Vitamin D 0mcg

Greek Gigantes Plaki (Baked Giant Beans)

Prep Time: 10 minutes | **Cooking Time:** 50 minutes | **Total Time:** 1 hour | **Serving:** 4 | **Cooking Difficulty:** Moderate

Ingredients:

- 1 cup dried giant beans (or large lima beans), soaked overnight
- 1 onion, diced
- 2 cloves garlic, minced
- 1 can (14 ounces) diced tomatoes
- 1/4 cup olive oil
- 1 tablespoon tomato paste
- 1 teaspoon dried oregano
- Salt and pepper, to taste
- Fresh parsley, for garnish (optional)

Instructions:

1. Preheat the oven to 350°F (175°C).
2. Drain and rinse the soaked beans. Boil in water for 30 minutes until tender, then drain and set aside.
3. In a skillet, heat olive oil over medium heat. Add the diced onion and garlic, and sauté for 5 minutes until softened.
4. Stir in the diced tomatoes, tomato paste, oregano, salt, and pepper. Simmer for 10 minutes until the sauce thickens.
5. In a baking dish, combine the cooked beans with the tomato sauce. Cover and bake for 30 minutes.
6. Garnish with fresh parsley and serve warm.

Nutritional Value:
Calories 380 | Fat 16g | Saturated Fat 2.5g | Cholesterol 0mg | Sodium 500mg | Carbohydrate 50g | Fiber 15g | Added Sugar 0g | Protein 12g | Calcium 100mg | Potassium 700mg | Iron 4mg | Vitamin D 0mcg

---

Japanese Natto Bowl

Prep Time: 5 minutes | **Cooking Time:** 0 minutes | **Total Time:** 5 minutes | **Serving:** 1 | **Cooking Difficulty:** Easy

Ingredients:

- 1 package (50g) natto (fermented soybeans)
- 1 cup cooked white or brown rice
- 1 green onion, sliced
- 1 teaspoon soy sauce (low sodium)
- 1/2 teaspoon mustard (optional)
- 1 teaspoon sesame seeds (optional)

Instructions:

1. Place the cooked rice in a bowl.
2. Open the natto package and mix it well to make it sticky. Add the mustard and soy sauce, and stir to combine.
3. Spoon the natto over the rice and garnish with sliced green onions and sesame seeds.
4. Serve immediately.

Nutritional Value:
Calories 290 | Fat 7g | Saturated Fat 1g | Cholesterol 0mg | Sodium 450mg | Carbohydrate 48g | Fiber 4g | Added Sugar 0g | Protein 12g | Calcium 50mg | Potassium 300mg | Iron 3mg | Vitamin D 0mcg

Thai Tempeh Curry

Prep Time: 10 minutes | **Cooking Time**: 20 minutes | **Total Time**: 30 minutes | **Serving**: 4 | **Cooking Difficulty**: Easy

Ingredients:

- 1 block (8 ounces) tempeh, cubed
- 1 can (14 ounces) coconut milk
- 2 tablespoons red curry paste
- 1/2 onion, sliced
- 1 red bell pepper, sliced
- 1 zucchini, sliced
- 1 tablespoon soy sauce (low sodium)
- 1 tablespoon olive oil
- 1 teaspoon ginger, minced
- 1 clove garlic, minced
- Fresh basil or cilantro for garnish
- Lime wedges, for serving
- Cooked jasmine rice, for serving

Instructions:

1. Heat olive oil in a large skillet over medium heat. Add the cubed tempeh and sauté for 5-7 minutes until golden brown. Remove and set aside.

2. In the same skillet, add the sliced onion, bell pepper, zucchini, ginger, and garlic. Sauté for 5 minutes until softened.

3. Stir in the red curry paste and cook for 1 minute until fragrant.

4. Add the coconut milk and soy sauce, and bring the mixture to a simmer. Cook for 5 minutes until the sauce thickens slightly.

5. Add the cooked tempeh back into the skillet and stir to combine.

6. Serve the curry over jasmine rice, garnished with fresh basil or cilantro and lime wedges.

Nutritional Value:

Calories 400 | Fat 24g | Saturated Fat 12g | Cholesterol 0mg | Sodium 450mg | Carbohydrate 35g | Fiber 8g | Added Sugar 0g | Protein 16g | Calcium 60mg | Potassium 500mg | Iron 3mg | Vitamin D 0mcg

Brazilian Black Bean Feijoada

Prep Time: 10 minutes | **Cooking Time**: 1 hour | **Total Time**: 1 hour 10 minutes | **Serving**: 4 | **Cooking Difficulty**: Moderate

Ingredients:

- 1 cup dried black beans, soaked overnight
- 1/2 pound smoked sausage, sliced (optional for authenticity)
- 1 onion, diced
- 2 cloves garlic, minced
- 1 bay leaf
- 1 tablespoon olive oil
- 1 teaspoon cumin
- 1/2 teaspoon smoked paprika
- Salt and pepper, to taste
- Fresh cilantro, for garnish
- Cooked white rice, for serving
- Orange slices, for serving (optional)

Instructions:

1. Drain and rinse the soaked black beans. In a large pot, cover the beans with water and bring to a boil. Reduce the heat and simmer for 45 minutes to 1 hour until tender.

2. In a separate skillet, heat olive oil over medium heat. Add the sausage slices (if using), onion,

and garlic, and sauté for 5-7 minutes until browned.

3. Add the cumin, smoked paprika, and bay leaf to the onion mixture, and stir to combine.

4. Once the beans are tender, add the onion and sausage mixture to the pot. Simmer for an additional 10 minutes, adjusting seasoning with salt and pepper.

5. Serve the feijoada with white rice, garnished with fresh cilantro and orange slices on the side.

Nutritional Value:

Calories 420 | Fat 18g | Saturated Fat 5g | Cholesterol 30mg | Sodium 600mg | Carbohydrate 50g | Fiber 14g | Added Sugar 0g | Protein 20g | Calcium 90mg | Potassium 700mg | Iron 4mg | Vitamin D 0mcg

Lebanese Mujaddara

Prep Time: 10 minutes | **Cooking Time:** 40 minutes | **Total Time:** 50 minutes | **Serving:** 4 | **Cooking Difficulty:** Easy

Ingredients:

- 1 cup lentils, rinsed

- 1/2 cup basmati rice

- 2 large onions, thinly sliced

- 1 tablespoon olive oil

- 1 teaspoon cumin

- 1/2 teaspoon cinnamon

- Salt and pepper, to taste

- Fresh parsley, for garnish

- Lemon wedges, for serving

Instructions:

1. In a pot, cover the lentils with water and bring to a boil. Simmer for 15-20 minutes until tender but still firm. Drain and set aside.

2. In a skillet, heat olive oil over medium heat. Add the sliced onions and cook for 15-20 minutes until caramelized and golden brown.

3. In the same pot used for the lentils, add the rice, cumin, cinnamon, salt, and pepper. Stir in 2 cups of water and bring to a boil. Reduce the heat, cover, and simmer for 15 minutes until the rice is cooked.

4. Stir the cooked lentils into the rice and mix well.

5. Serve the mujaddara topped with caramelized onions, garnished with parsley, and lemon wedges on the side.

Nutritional Value:

Calories 350 | Fat 8g | Saturated Fat 1g | Cholesterol 0mg | Sodium 200mg | Carbohydrate 60g | Fiber 14g | Added Sugar 0g | Protein 12g | Calcium 60mg | Potassium 600mg | Iron 3.5mg | Vitamin D 0mcg

Turkish Red Lentil Soup

Prep Time: 10 minutes | **Cooking Time:** 30 minutes | **Total Time:** 40 minutes | **Serving:** 4 | **Cooking Difficulty:** Easy

Ingredients:

- 1 cup red lentils, rinsed

- 1 onion, diced

- 2 carrots, diced

- 2 cloves garlic, minced

- 1 tablespoon tomato paste

- 1 teaspoon cumin

- 1 teaspoon paprika

- 1/4 teaspoon chili flakes (optional)

- 4 cups vegetable broth

- 1 tablespoon olive oil

- Salt and pepper, to taste

- Fresh lemon wedges, for serving

Instructions:

1. Heat olive oil in a large pot over medium heat. Add the diced onion, carrots, and garlic, and sauté for 5-7 minutes until softened.

2. Stir in the tomato paste, cumin, paprika, and chili flakes. Cook for 1-2 minutes until fragrant.

3. Add the rinsed lentils and vegetable broth. Bring to a boil, then reduce heat and simmer for 20-25 minutes until the lentils are tender.

4. Using an immersion blender, blend the soup until smooth (optional, leave chunky if preferred).

5. Season with salt and pepper, and serve with fresh lemon wedges.

Nutritional Value:

Calories 250 | Fat 7g | Saturated Fat 1g | Cholesterol 0mg | Sodium 500mg | Carbohydrate 40g | Fiber 12g | Added Sugar 0g | Protein 14g | Calcium 60mg | Potassium 650mg | Iron 3mg | Vitamin D 0mcg

Korean Doenjang Stew (Doenjang Jjigae)

Prep Time: 10 minutes | **Cooking Time**: 25 minutes | **Total Time**: 35 minutes | **Serving**: 4 | **Cooking Difficulty**: Moderate

Ingredients:

- 2 tablespoons doenjang (Korean fermented soybean paste)

- 1/2 block (7 ounces) tofu, cubed

- 1 zucchini, sliced

- 1 small potato, diced

- 1 onion, sliced

- 2 cloves garlic, minced

- 1 teaspoon gochugaru (Korean chili flakes, optional)

- 4 cups vegetable or dashi broth

- 1 tablespoon sesame oil

- 1 green onion, sliced, for garnish

- Cooked rice, for serving

Instructions:

1. In a pot, heat sesame oil over medium heat. Add the minced garlic and sliced onion, and sauté for 2-3 minutes until softened.

2. Add the doenjang paste and stir well. Cook for 1-2 minutes until fragrant.

3. Pour in the broth and bring to a boil. Add the diced potato and zucchini, and simmer for 10 minutes until the vegetables are tender.

4. Stir in the tofu and gochugaru (if using), and simmer for an additional 5 minutes.

5. Garnish with sliced green onions and serve with cooked rice.

Nutritional Value:

Calories 280 | Fat 12g | Saturated Fat 2g | Cholesterol 0mg | Sodium 750mg | Carbohydrate 30g | Fiber 6g | Added Sugar 0g | Protein 14g | Calcium 100mg | Potassium 600mg | Iron 3mg | Vitamin D 0mcg

Lentil and Sausage Rice Pot

Prep Time: 10 minutes | **Cooking Time:** 30 minutes | **Total Time:** 40 minutes | **Serving:** 4 | **Cooking Difficulty:** Easy

Ingredients:

- 1/2 pound sausage (chicken, turkey, or plant-based), sliced
- 1 cup lentils, rinsed
- 1 cup basmati rice
- 1 onion, diced
- 2 cloves garlic, minced
- 1 teaspoon cumin
- 1 teaspoon smoked paprika
- 3 cups chicken or vegetable broth
- 1 tablespoon olive oil
- Salt and pepper, to taste
- Fresh parsley, for garnish

Instructions:

1. Heat olive oil in a large pot over medium heat. Add the sausage slices and cook until browned, about 5-7 minutes. Remove and set aside.

2. In the same pot, add the onion and garlic, and sauté for 3-5 minutes until softened.

3. Stir in the cumin, smoked paprika, lentils, and rice. Cook for 1-2 minutes to toast the rice slightly.

4. Add the broth, bring to a boil, and reduce heat to low. Cover and simmer for 25-30 minutes until the lentils and rice are tender and the liquid is absorbed.

5. Stir the cooked sausage back into the pot and season with salt and pepper.

6. Garnish with fresh parsley and serve warm.

Nutritional Value:

Calories 420 | Fat 12g | Saturated Fat 3g | Cholesterol 30mg | Sodium 600mg | Carbohydrate 60g | Fiber 12g | Added Sugar 0g | Protein 20g | Calcium 60mg | Potassium 700mg | Iron 4mg | Vitamin D 0mcg

Three Bean Cajun Jambalaya

Prep Time: 10 minutes | **Cooking Time:** 30 minutes | **Total Time:** 40 minutes | **Serving:** 4 | **Cooking Difficulty:** Easy

Ingredients:

- 1/2 cup black beans, drained and rinsed
- 1/2 cup kidney beans, drained and rinsed
- 1/2 cup pinto beans, drained and rinsed
- 1 cup basmati rice
- 1/2 onion, diced
- 1 bell pepper, diced
- 2 cloves garlic, minced
- 1 tablespoon Cajun seasoning
- 2 cups vegetable broth
- 1 tablespoon olive oil
- Salt and pepper, to taste
- Fresh parsley, for garnish

Instructions:

1. Heat olive oil in a large skillet over medium heat. Add the onion, bell pepper, and garlic, and sauté for 5 minutes until softened.

2. Stir in the Cajun seasoning, black beans, kidney beans, pinto beans, and rice. Cook for 1-2 minutes to toast the rice slightly.

3. Add the vegetable broth, bring to a boil, and reduce heat to low. Cover and simmer for 20-25 minutes until the rice is tender and the liquid is absorbed.

4. Season with salt and pepper, garnish with fresh parsley, and serve warm.

Nutritional Value:

Calories 350 | Fat 6g | Saturated Fat 1g | Cholesterol 0mg | Sodium 500mg | Carbohydrate 65g | Fiber 15g | Added Sugar 0g | Protein 14g | Calcium 80mg | Potassium 700mg | Iron 3mg | Vitamin D 0mcg

Chickpea Quinoa Pilaf

Prep Time: 10 minutes | **Cooking Time**: 20 minutes | **Total Time**: 30 minutes | **Serving**: 4 | **Cooking Difficulty**: Easy

Ingredients:

- 1 cup quinoa, rinsed
- 1 can (15 ounces) chickpeas, drained and rinsed
- 1/4 cup dried cranberries (optional)
- 1/4 cup slivered almonds (optional)
- 1/2 onion, diced
- 2 cloves garlic, minced
- 1 tablespoon olive oil
- 2 cups vegetable broth
- 1/2 teaspoon cumin
- Salt and pepper, to taste
- Fresh parsley, for garnish

Instructions:

1. Heat olive oil in a large pot over medium heat. Add the onion and garlic, and sauté for 5 minutes until softened.

2. Stir in the cumin and quinoa, and cook for 1-2 minutes to toast the quinoa slightly.

3. Add the vegetable broth and bring to a boil. Reduce heat, cover, and simmer for 15 minutes until the quinoa is cooked.

4. Stir in the chickpeas, dried cranberries, and slivered almonds. Season with salt and pepper.

5. Garnish with fresh parsley and serve warm.

Nutritional Value:

Calories 300 | Fat 10g | Saturated Fat 1.5g | Cholesterol 0mg | Sodium 400mg | Carbohydrate 45g | Fiber 10g | Added Sugar 5g | Protein 12g | Calcium 60mg | Potassium 600mg | Iron 3mg | Vitamin D 0mcg

Black Bean Southwest Skillet

Prep Time: 10 minutes | **Cooking Time**: 15 minutes | **Total Time**: 25 minutes | **Serving**: 4 | **Cooking Difficulty**: Easy

Ingredients:

- 1 can (15 ounces) black beans, drained and rinsed
- 1/2 cup corn kernels (fresh or frozen)
- 1/2 cup diced tomatoes
- 1/4 cup bell peppers, diced
- 1/2 onion, diced
- 2 cloves garlic, minced
- 1 teaspoon cumin
- 1 teaspoon chili powder
- 1 tablespoon olive oil
- Salt and pepper, to taste
- Fresh cilantro, for garnish

Instructions:

1. Heat olive oil in a large skillet over medium heat. Add the onion, bell pepper, and garlic, and sauté for 5 minutes until softened.

2. Stir in the cumin, chili powder, black beans, corn, and diced tomatoes. Cook for 5-7 minutes until heated through.

3. Season with salt and pepper, and garnish with fresh cilantro before serving.

Nutritional Value:

Calories 280 | Fat 8g | Saturated Fat 1g | Cholesterol 0mg | Sodium 400mg | Carbohydrate 40g | Fiber 12g | Added Sugar 0g | Protein 10g | Calcium 50mg | Potassium 600mg | Iron 3mg | Vitamin D 0mcg

White Bean Tuscan Stew

Prep Time: 10 minutes | **Cooking Time:** 30 minutes | **Total Time:** 40 minutes | **Serving:** 4 | **Cooking Difficulty:** Easy

Ingredients:

- 1 can (15 ounces) white beans, drained and rinsed
- 1/2 cup diced tomatoes
- 1/4 cup carrots, diced
- 1/4 cup celery, diced
- 1 onion, diced
- 2 cloves garlic, minced
- 1 tablespoon olive oil
- 4 cups vegetable broth
- 1 teaspoon dried thyme
- 1/2 teaspoon rosemary
- Salt and pepper, to taste
- Fresh spinach (optional), for serving
- Fresh basil, for garnish

Instructions:

1. Heat olive oil in a large pot over medium heat. Add the onion, carrots, celery, and garlic, and sauté for 5 minutes until softened.

2. Stir in the thyme, rosemary, white beans, and diced tomatoes. Add the vegetable broth and bring to a boil.

3. Reduce heat, cover, and simmer for 20 minutes until the vegetables are tender.

4. Season with salt and pepper, stir in fresh spinach if desired, and garnish with fresh basil before serving.

Nutritional Value:

Calories 300 | Fat 8g | Saturated Fat 1g | Cholesterol 0mg | Sodium 500mg | Carbohydrate 45g | Fiber 12g | Added Sugar 0g | Protein 12g | Calcium 80mg | Potassium 700mg | Iron 3mg | Vitamin D 0mcg

Red Lentil Curry Rice

Prep Time: 10 minutes | **Cooking Time:** 25 minutes | **Total Time:** 35 minutes | **Serving:** 4 | **Cooking Difficulty:** Easy

Ingredients:

- 1 cup red lentils, rinsed
- 1 cup basmati rice
- 1/2 onion, diced
- 2 cloves garlic, minced
- 1 tablespoon curry powder
- 1 teaspoon turmeric
- 1 teaspoon cumin
- 1 tablespoon olive oil
- 3 cups vegetable broth
- Salt and pepper, to taste
- Fresh cilantro, for garnish (optional)

Instructions:

1. Heat olive oil in a large pot over medium heat. Add the diced onion and garlic, and sauté for 3-5 minutes until softened.

2. Stir in the curry powder, turmeric, cumin, and rice. Cook for 1-2 minutes to toast the rice.

3. Add the red lentils and vegetable broth. Bring to a boil, then reduce heat, cover, and simmer for 20-25 minutes until the rice and lentils are tender and the liquid is absorbed.

4. Season with salt and pepper, and garnish with fresh cilantro if desired. Serve warm.

Nutritional Value:
Calories 350 | Fat 8g | Saturated Fat 1g | Cholesterol 0mg | Sodium 400mg | Carbohydrate 60g | Fiber 12g | Added Sugar 0g | Protein 15g | Calcium 60mg | Potassium 650mg | Iron 3mg | Vitamin D 0mcg

Navy Bean Irish Coddle

Prep Time: 10 minutes | **Cooking Time**: 1 hour | **Total Time**: 1 hour 10 minutes | **Serving**: 4 | **Cooking Difficulty**: Moderate

Ingredients:

- 1 can (15 ounces) navy beans, drained and rinsed
- 1/2 pound sausages (pork, turkey, or plant-based), sliced
- 1/2 pound potatoes, diced
- 1 onion, sliced
- 2 carrots, sliced
- 2 cloves garlic, minced
- 1 tablespoon olive oil
- 3 cups vegetable broth
- 1 bay leaf
- Salt and pepper, to taste
- Fresh parsley, for garnish

Instructions:

1. Heat olive oil in a large pot over medium heat. Add the sliced sausage and cook until browned, about 5-7 minutes. Remove and set aside.

2. In the same pot, add the onions, carrots, and garlic, and sauté for 5 minutes until softened.

3. Add the diced potatoes, navy beans, vegetable broth, and bay leaf. Bring to a boil, then reduce heat and simmer for 40-45 minutes until the potatoes are tender.

4. Return the sausage to the pot and simmer for an additional 5-10 minutes.

5. Season with salt and pepper, garnish with fresh parsley, and serve warm.

Nutritional Value:
Calories 400 | Fat 14g | Saturated Fat 4g | Cholesterol 30mg | Sodium 600mg | Carbohydrate 50g | Fiber 10g | Added Sugar 0g | Protein 20g | Calcium 80mg | Potassium 800mg | Iron 3.5mg | Vitamin D 0mcg

Mung Bean Asian Rice Bowl

Prep Time: 10 minutes | **Cooking Time**: 25 minutes | **Total Time**: 35 minutes | **Serving**: 4 | **Cooking Difficulty**: Easy

Ingredients:

- 1 cup cooked mung beans
- 1 cup jasmine rice
- 1/4 cup shredded carrots
- 1/4 cup bell peppers, sliced
- 1 tablespoon soy sauce (low sodium)
- 1 tablespoon sesame oil
- 1 teaspoon rice vinegar
- 2 cloves garlic, minced
- Sesame seeds (optional, for garnish)

Instructions:

1. Cook jasmine rice according to package instructions and set aside.

2. In a large skillet, heat sesame oil over medium heat. Add the garlic, shredded carrots, and bell peppers, and sauté for 3-5 minutes until softened.

3. Stir in the cooked mung beans, soy sauce, and rice vinegar. Cook for 2-3 minutes until the mung beans are heated through.

4. Serve the mung bean mixture over jasmine rice, garnished with sesame seeds if desired.

Nutritional Value:

Calories 300 | Fat 8g | Saturated Fat 1g | Cholesterol 0mg | Sodium 400mg | Carbohydrate 50g | Fiber 6g | Added Sugar 0g | Protein 10g | Calcium 50mg | Potassium 450mg | Iron 2mg | Vitamin D 0mcg

Lima Bean Southern Style Pot

Prep Time: 10 minutes | **Cooking Time:** 45 minutes | **Total Time:** 55 minutes | **Serving:** 4 | **Cooking Difficulty:** Moderate

Ingredients:

- 1 cup dried lima beans, soaked overnight
- 1/2 pound smoked sausage or ham (optional), diced
- 1 onion, diced
- 2 cloves garlic, minced
- 1 teaspoon paprika
- 1/2 teaspoon cayenne pepper (optional)
- 1 tablespoon olive oil
- 4 cups vegetable or chicken broth
- Salt and pepper, to taste
- Fresh parsley, for garnish

Instructions:

1. Heat olive oil in a large pot over medium heat. Add the diced sausage or ham (if using) and cook until browned. Remove and set aside.

2. In the same pot, add the diced onion and garlic, and sauté for 5 minutes until softened.

3. Add the soaked lima beans, paprika, cayenne pepper, and broth. Bring to a boil, then reduce

heat and simmer for 40-45 minutes until the beans are tender.

4. Stir in the cooked sausage or ham, season with salt and pepper, and cook for an additional 5 minutes.

5. Garnish with fresh parsley and serve warm.

Nutritional Value:

Calories 350 | Fat 10g | Saturated Fat 3g | Cholesterol 25mg | Sodium 500mg | Carbohydrate 45g | Fiber 12g | Added Sugar 0g | Protein 20g | Calcium 70mg | Potassium 700mg | Iron 3mg | Vitamin D 0mcg

Split Pea Dutch Oven Stew

Prep Time: 10 minutes | **Cooking Time:** 1 hour | **Total Time:** 1 hour 10 minutes | **Serving:** 4 | **Cooking Difficulty:** Moderate

Ingredients:

- 1 cup dried split peas, rinsed
- 1/2 cup diced carrots
- 1/2 cup diced celery
- 1 onion, diced
- 2 cloves garlic, minced
- 4 cups vegetable broth
- 1 bay leaf
- 1 tablespoon olive oil
- 1 teaspoon thyme
- Salt and pepper, to taste
- Fresh parsley, for garnish

Instructions:

1. Preheat the oven to 350°F (175°C).

2. In a Dutch oven, heat olive oil over medium heat. Add the onion, carrots, celery, and garlic, and sauté for 5-7 minutes until softened.

3. Stir in the split peas, thyme, vegetable broth, and bay leaf. Bring to a boil.

4. Cover the Dutch oven and transfer to the preheated oven. Bake for 1 hour, or until the peas are tender.

5. Remove the bay leaf, season with salt and pepper, and garnish with fresh parsley before serving.

Nutritional Value:
Calories 320 | Fat 8g | Saturated Fat 1g | Cholesterol 0mg | Sodium 450mg | Carbohydrate 50g | Fiber 15g | Added Sugar 0g | Protein 15g | Calcium 60mg | Potassium 700mg | Iron 3mg | Vitamin D 0mcg

Protein-Rich Baked Goods

Black Bean Breakfast Muffins

Prep Time: 10 minutes | **Cooking Time**: 20 minutes | **Total Time**: 30 minutes | **Serving**: 12 muffins | **Cooking Difficulty**: Easy

Ingredients:

- 1 can (15 ounces) black beans, drained and rinsed
- 1/4 cup cocoa powder
- 1/4 cup rolled oats
- 1/4 cup honey or maple syrup
- 2 eggs
- 1/4 cup coconut oil, melted
- 1 teaspoon vanilla extract
- 1 teaspoon baking powder
- 1/2 teaspoon baking soda
- Pinch of salt
- 1/4 cup dark chocolate chips (optional)

Instructions:

1. Preheat the oven to 350°F (175°C) and line a muffin tin with paper liners.
2. In a blender or food processor, combine the black beans, cocoa powder, oats, honey, eggs, coconut oil, vanilla extract, baking powder, baking soda, and salt. Blend until smooth.
3. Stir in the dark chocolate chips if using.
4. Divide the batter evenly among the muffin cups.
5. Bake for 18-20 minutes, or until a toothpick inserted into the center comes out clean.
6. Let the muffins cool before serving.

Nutritional Value:

Calories 120 | Fat 7g | Saturated Fat 3g | Cholesterol 30mg | Sodium 150mg | Carbohydrate 15g | Fiber 4g | Added Sugar 6g | Protein 5g | Calcium 40mg | Potassium 150mg | Iron 1.5mg | Vitamin D 0mcg

Chickpea Flour Bread

Prep Time: 10 minutes | **Cooking Time**: 35 minutes | **Total Time**: 45 minutes | **Serving**: 8 slices | **Cooking Difficulty**: Easy

Ingredients:

- 1 1/2 cups chickpea flour (gram flour)
- 1 teaspoon baking powder
- 1/2 teaspoon salt
- 1 tablespoon olive oil
- 1 tablespoon apple cider vinegar
- 1 cup water
- Optional: herbs (thyme, rosemary) for added flavor

Instructions:

1. Preheat the oven to 350°F (175°C) and grease a loaf pan.
2. In a large bowl, whisk together chickpea flour, baking powder, salt, and any optional herbs.
3. Add the olive oil, apple cider vinegar, and water, and mix until you have a smooth batter.
4. Pour the batter into the prepared loaf pan and smooth the top.

5. Bake for 30-35 minutes, or until a toothpick inserted in the center comes out clean.

6. Let the bread cool before slicing and serving.

Nutritional Value:
Calories 110 | Fat 3g | Saturated Fat 0.5g | Cholesterol 0mg | Sodium 250mg | Carbohydrate 16g | Fiber 3g | Added Sugar 0g | Protein 6g | Calcium 30mg | Potassium 180mg | Iron 2mg | Vitamin D 0mcg

Lentil Protein Scones

Prep Time: 15 minutes | **Cooking Time:** 20 minutes | **Total Time:** 35 minutes | **Serving:** 8 scones | **Cooking Difficulty:** Moderate

Ingredients:

- 1 cup cooked red lentils, mashed
- 1 1/2 cups whole wheat flour
- 1/4 cup rolled oats
- 1/4 cup coconut oil, chilled and cubed
- 2 tablespoons honey or maple syrup
- 2 teaspoons baking powder
- 1/4 teaspoon salt
- 1/2 cup almond milk (or dairy-free alternative)

Instructions:

1. Preheat the oven to 375°F (190°C) and line a baking sheet with parchment paper.

2. In a large bowl, combine the flour, oats, baking powder, and salt.

3. Add the cubed coconut oil and mix with your hands or a pastry cutter until the mixture resembles coarse crumbs.

4. Stir in the mashed lentils, honey, and almond milk. Mix until just combined (don't overmix).

5. Turn the dough onto a floured surface, form into a round disk, and cut into 8 wedges.

6. Place the scones on the prepared baking sheet and bake for 18-20 minutes, or until golden.

7. Let cool slightly before serving.

Nutritional Value:
Calories 180 | Fat 8g | Saturated Fat 5g | Cholesterol 0mg | Sodium 180mg | Carbohydrate 25g | Fiber 4g | Added Sugar 4g | Protein 6g | Calcium 40mg | Potassium 200mg | Iron 2mg | Vitamin D 0mcg

Quinoa Protein Bars

Prep Time: 10 minutes | **Cooking Time:** 0 minutes | **Total Time:** 10 minutes (plus chilling time) | **Serving:** 8 bars | **Cooking Difficulty:** Easy

Ingredients:

- 1/2 cup cooked quinoa
- 1/2 cup rolled oats
- 1/4 cup almond butter or peanut butter
- 1/4 cup honey or maple syrup
- 1/4 cup protein powder (optional)
- 1/4 cup dark chocolate chips
- 1/2 teaspoon vanilla extract
- Pinch of salt

Instructions:

1. In a large bowl, mix the cooked quinoa, oats, almond butter, honey, protein powder (if using), vanilla extract, and salt until well combined.

2. Stir in the dark chocolate chips.

3. Press the mixture firmly into an 8x8-inch baking dish lined with parchment paper.

4. Refrigerate for at least 1 hour to firm up.

5. Slice into bars and store in the refrigerator.

Nutritional Value:
Calories 220 | Fat 10g | Saturated Fat 2.5g | Cholesterol 0mg | Sodium 60mg | Carbohydrate 26g | Fiber 4g | Added Sugar 10g | Protein 8g | Calcium 40mg | Potassium 200mg | Iron 2mg | Vitamin D 0mcg

Bean Flour Pizza Crust

Prep Time: 10 minutes | **Cooking Time:** 20 minutes | **Total Time:** 30 minutes | **Serving:** 1 pizza crust (8 slices) | **Cooking Difficulty:** Moderate

Ingredients:

- 1 1/2 cups chickpea flour or other bean flour (such as lentil or black bean flour)
- 1 teaspoon baking powder
- 1/2 teaspoon salt
- 1 tablespoon olive oil
- 1/2 cup water (add more if needed)
- Optional: dried herbs (oregano, basil) for added flavor

Instructions:

1. Preheat the oven to 400°F (200°C) and line a baking sheet with parchment paper.
2. In a bowl, whisk together the bean flour, baking powder, salt, and any optional herbs.
3. Add the olive oil and water, and stir until a dough forms. It should be firm but pliable; add more water if needed.
4. Place the dough on the prepared baking sheet and press or roll it out into a thin circle or rectangle.
5. Bake for 10 minutes, then remove from the oven and add your desired toppings.
6. Return to the oven and bake for an additional 10-12 minutes until the crust is golden and the toppings are cooked.

7. Slice and serve.

Nutritional Value:
Calories 110 (per slice, without toppings) | Fat 3g | Saturated Fat 0.5g | Cholesterol 0mg | Sodium 150mg | Carbohydrate 15g | Fiber 4g | Added Sugar 0g | Protein 6g | Calcium 40mg | Potassium 180mg | Iron 2mg | Vitamin D 0mcg

High-Protein Banana Bread

Prep Time: 10 minutes | **Cooking Time:** 50 minutes | **Total Time:** 1 hour | **Serving:** 8 slices | **Cooking Difficulty:** Easy

Ingredients:

- 3 ripe bananas, mashed
- 1/2 cup almond flour
- 1/2 cup chickpea flour
- 1/4 cup protein powder (optional)
- 2 eggs
- 1/4 cup almond butter or peanut butter
- 2 tablespoons honey or maple syrup
- 1 teaspoon vanilla extract
- 1 teaspoon baking powder
- 1/2 teaspoon cinnamon
- Pinch of salt

Instructions:

1. Preheat the oven to 350°F (175°C) and grease a loaf pan.
2. In a large bowl, mix together the mashed bananas, eggs, almond butter, honey, and vanilla extract until well combined.
3. In a separate bowl, whisk together the almond flour, chickpea flour, protein powder (if using), baking powder, cinnamon, and salt.

4. Combine the wet and dry ingredients and mix until just combined.

5. Pour the batter into the prepared loaf pan and smooth the top.

6. Bake for 45-50 minutes, or until a toothpick inserted in the center comes out clean.

7. Allow the banana bread to cool before slicing.

Nutritional Value:
Calories 220 | Fat 10g | Saturated Fat 1.5g | Cholesterol 50mg | Sodium 150mg | Carbohydrate 25g | Fiber 4g | Added Sugar 6g | Protein 9g | Calcium 40mg | Potassium 300mg | Iron 1.5mg | Vitamin D 0mcg

Tempeh "Meat" Loaf

Prep Time: 15 minutes | **Cooking Time:** 45 minutes | **Total Time:** 1 hour | **Serving:** 6 | **Cooking Difficulty:** Moderate

Ingredients:

- 1 block (8 ounces) tempeh, crumbled
- 1/2 cup cooked lentils
- 1/2 cup rolled oats
- 1/4 cup breadcrumbs (whole wheat or gluten-free)
- 1/4 cup tomato paste
- 1/4 cup onion, finely chopped
- 1 clove garlic, minced
- 1 tablespoon soy sauce (low sodium)
- 1 tablespoon olive oil
- 1 teaspoon dried thyme
- 1 teaspoon smoked paprika
- Salt and pepper, to taste

Instructions:

1. Preheat the oven to 350°F (175°C) and grease a loaf pan.

2. In a large bowl, combine the crumbled tempeh, cooked lentils, oats, breadcrumbs, onion, garlic, tomato paste, soy sauce, olive oil, thyme, smoked paprika, salt, and pepper.

3. Mix until well combined and form into a loaf shape in the prepared loaf pan.

4. Bake for 40-45 minutes, until the loaf is firm and golden on top.

5. Let the loaf cool slightly before slicing and serving.

Nutritional Value:
Calories 240 | Fat 9g | Saturated Fat 1.5g | Cholesterol 0mg | Sodium 300mg | Carbohydrate 30g | Fiber 7g | Added Sugar 2g | Protein 14g | Calcium 50mg | Potassium 450mg | Iron 3mg | Vitamin D 0mcg

Legume-Based Coffee Cake

Prep Time: 15 minutes | **Cooking Time:** 30 minutes | **Total Time:** 45 minutes | **Serving:** 8 slices | **Cooking Difficulty:** Moderate

Ingredients:

- 1 cup chickpea flour
- 1/2 cup almond flour
- 1/4 cup coconut oil, melted
- 1/4 cup honey or maple syrup
- 2 eggs
- 1/4 cup almond milk (or dairy-free milk)
- 1 teaspoon vanilla extract
- 1 teaspoon baking powder
- 1/2 teaspoon cinnamon
- Pinch of salt

Topping:

- 2 tablespoons coconut sugar

- 2 tablespoons almond flour

- 1 teaspoon cinnamon

- 1 tablespoon coconut oil, melted

Instructions:

1. Preheat the oven to 350°F (175°C) and grease a baking dish.

2. In a large bowl, mix together the chickpea flour, almond flour, coconut oil, honey, eggs, almond milk, vanilla extract, baking powder, cinnamon, and salt until smooth.

3. Pour the batter into the prepared baking dish and smooth the top.

4. In a small bowl, mix the topping ingredients (coconut sugar, almond flour, cinnamon, and melted coconut oil) and sprinkle over the batter.

5. Bake for 25-30 minutes, or until a toothpick inserted in the center comes out clean.

6. Allow the cake to cool before serving.

Nutritional Value:
Calories 240 | Fat 12g | Saturated Fat 5g | Cholesterol 40mg | Sodium 100mg | Carbohydrate 28g | Fiber 5g | Added Sugar 8g | Protein 6g | Calcium 40mg | Potassium 200mg | Iron 1.5mg | Vitamin D 0mcg

Bean and Seed Crackers

Prep Time: 10 minutes | **Cooking Time:** 20 minutes | **Total Time:** 30 minutes | **Serving:** 20 crackers | **Cooking Difficulty:** Easy

Ingredients:

- 1/2 cup chickpea flour

- 1/4 cup sunflower seeds

- 1/4 cup flaxseeds

- 2 tablespoons sesame seeds

- 1 tablespoon olive oil

- 1/2 teaspoon garlic powder

- 1/4 teaspoon salt

- 1/4 cup water (add more if needed)

Instructions:

1. Preheat the oven to 350°F (175°C) and line a baking sheet with parchment paper.

2. In a large bowl, mix together the chickpea flour, sunflower seeds, flaxseeds, sesame seeds, garlic powder, and salt.

3. Add the olive oil and water, and stir until a dough forms.

4. Roll the dough between two sheets of parchment paper until about 1/8-inch thick. Cut into squares or shapes.

5. Place the crackers on the prepared baking sheet and bake for 15-20 minutes, until golden and crispy.

6. Let cool before serving.

Nutritional Value:
Calories 70 | Fat 4g | Saturated Fat 0.5g | Cholesterol 0mg | Sodium 80mg | Carbohydrate 6g | Fiber 2g | Added Sugar 0g | Protein 3g | Calcium 20mg | Potassium 100mg | Iron 0.5mg | Vitamin D 0mcg

Protein Power Biscuits

Prep Time: 10 minutes | **Cooking Time**: 15 minutes | **Total Time**: 25 minutes | **Serving**: 8 biscuits | **Cooking Difficulty**: Easy

Ingredients:

- 1 cup chickpea flour
- 1/4 cup almond flour
- 1/4 cup protein powder (optional)
- 1/4 cup coconut oil, chilled and cubed
- 1/4 cup almond milk (or dairy-free milk)
- 1 tablespoon baking powder
- 1/4 teaspoon salt
- 1 tablespoon honey (optional, for sweetness)

Instructions:

1. Preheat the oven to 375°F (190°C) and line a baking sheet with parchment paper.
2. In a large bowl, whisk together the chickpea flour, almond flour, protein powder, baking powder, and salt.
3. Add the cubed coconut oil and mix with your hands or a pastry cutter until the mixture resembles coarse crumbs.
4. Stir in the almond milk and honey (if using) until a dough forms.
5. Drop spoonfuls of dough onto the prepared baking sheet and bake for 12-15 minutes, or until golden brown.
6. Let cool slightly before serving.

Nutritional Value:
Calories 160 | Fat 9g | Saturated Fat 5g | Cholesterol 0mg | Sodium 200mg | Carbohydrate 15g | Fiber 4g | Added Sugar 2g | Protein 6g | Calcium 50mg | Potassium 150mg | Iron 1mg | Vitamin D 0mcg

Plant-Based Power Meals

Tempeh Black Bean Power Plate

Prep Time: 10 minutes | **Cooking Time:** 15 minutes | **Total Time:** 25 minutes | **Serving:** 2 | **Cooking Difficulty:** Easy

Ingredients:

- 1 block (8 ounces) tempeh, cubed
- 1/2 cup black beans, drained and rinsed
- 1/4 cup corn kernels (fresh or frozen)
- 1/4 cup cherry tomatoes, halved
- 1/2 avocado, sliced
- 1 tablespoon olive oil
- 1 tablespoon soy sauce (low sodium)
- 1 teaspoon cumin
- Salt and pepper, to taste
- Fresh cilantro, for garnish

Instructions:

1. Heat olive oil in a skillet over medium heat. Add the cubed tempeh and cook for 5-7 minutes, turning occasionally, until golden brown.
2. Stir in the soy sauce, cumin, salt, and pepper. Cook for another 1-2 minutes.
3. In a serving plate, arrange the black beans, corn, cherry tomatoes, avocado slices, and cooked tempeh.
4. Garnish with fresh cilantro and serve immediately.

Nutritional Value:

Calories 380 | Fat 18g | Saturated Fat 2.5g | Cholesterol 0mg | Sodium 400mg | Carbohydrate 35g | Fiber 12g | Added Sugar 0g | Protein 20g | Calcium 80mg | Potassium 600mg | Iron 3mg | Vitamin D 0mcg

Chickpea Quinoa Buddha Bowl

Prep Time: 10 minutes | **Cooking Time:** 15 minutes | **Total Time:** 25 minutes | **Serving:** 2 | **Cooking Difficulty:** Easy

Ingredients:

- 1/2 cup quinoa, rinsed
- 1/2 cup cooked chickpeas
- 1/4 cup diced cucumber
- 1/4 cup shredded carrots
- 1/4 cup cherry tomatoes, halved
- 1 tablespoon tahini
- 1 tablespoon lemon juice
- 1 tablespoon olive oil
- Salt and pepper, to taste
- Fresh parsley, for garnish

Instructions:

1. Cook the quinoa according to package instructions. Set aside.
2. In a serving bowl, layer the cooked quinoa, chickpeas, cucumber, shredded carrots, and cherry tomatoes.
3. In a small bowl, whisk together the tahini, lemon juice, olive oil, salt, and pepper.

4. Drizzle the dressing over the Buddha bowl and toss lightly.

5. Garnish with fresh parsley and serve immediately.

Nutritional Value:
Calories 350 | Fat 14g | Saturated Fat 2g | Cholesterol 0mg | Sodium 220mg | Carbohydrate 50g | Fiber 10g | Added Sugar 0g | Protein 12g | Calcium 60mg | Potassium 550mg | Iron 3mg | Vitamin D 0mcg

Lentil Vegetable Grain Bowl

Prep Time: 10 minutes | **Cooking Time:** 20 minutes | **Total Time:** 30 minutes | **Serving:** 2 | **Cooking Difficulty:** Easy

Ingredients:

- 1/2 cup cooked lentils
- 1/2 cup farro or brown rice
- 1/4 cup roasted sweet potatoes
- 1/4 cup sautéed spinach
- 1/4 cup diced bell peppers
- 1 tablespoon olive oil
- 1 teaspoon balsamic vinegar
- Salt and pepper, to taste
- Fresh basil, for garnish

Instructions:

1. Cook the farro or brown rice according to package instructions. Set aside.

2. In a serving bowl, layer the cooked lentils, farro, roasted sweet potatoes, sautéed spinach, and diced bell peppers.

3. Drizzle olive oil and balsamic vinegar over the bowl, and season with salt and pepper.

4. Garnish with fresh basil and serve warm.

Nutritional Value:
Calories 400 | Fat 12g | Saturated Fat 1.5g | Cholesterol 0mg | Sodium 250mg | Carbohydrate 60g | Fiber 12g | Added Sugar 0g | Protein 15g | Calcium 80mg | Potassium 650mg | Iron 4mg | Vitamin D 0mcg

Three Bean Protein Platter

Prep Time: 10 minutes | **Cooking Time:** 0 minutes | **Total Time:** 10 minutes | **Serving:** 2 | **Cooking Difficulty:** Easy

Ingredients:

- 1/2 cup black beans, drained and rinsed
- 1/2 cup kidney beans, drained and rinsed
- 1/2 cup chickpeas, drained and rinsed
- 1/4 cup diced cucumber
- 1/4 cup diced tomatoes
- 1 tablespoon olive oil
- 1 tablespoon lemon juice
- Salt and pepper, to taste
- Fresh cilantro, for garnish

Instructions:

1. In a large bowl, combine the black beans, kidney beans, chickpeas, cucumber, and tomatoes.

2. Drizzle with olive oil and lemon juice, and season with salt and pepper.

3. Toss the mixture gently and garnish with fresh cilantro.

4. Serve immediately as a light meal or snack.

Nutritional Value:
Calories 300 | Fat 10g | Saturated Fat 1.5g | Cholesterol 0mg | Sodium 200mg | Carbohydrate 45g | Fiber 12g | Added Sugar 0g | Protein 15g | Calcium 80mg | Potassium 700mg | Iron 4mg | Vitamin D 0mcg

Edamame Rice Power Bowl

Prep Time: 10 minutes | **Cooking Time**: 15 minutes | **Total Time**: 25 minutes | **Serving**: 2 | **Cooking Difficulty**: Easy

Ingredients:

- 1/2 cup cooked brown rice
- 1/2 cup shelled edamame
- 1/4 cup shredded carrots
- 1/4 cup diced cucumbers
- 1 tablespoon soy sauce (low sodium)
- 1 tablespoon sesame oil
- 1 teaspoon rice vinegar
- Sesame seeds (optional, for garnish)

Instructions:

1. Cook the brown rice according to package instructions and set aside.
2. Steam the edamame until tender, then drain.
3. In a serving bowl, layer the cooked brown rice, edamame, shredded carrots, and diced cucumbers.
4. In a small bowl, whisk together the soy sauce, sesame oil, and rice vinegar.
5. Drizzle the dressing over the bowl, toss lightly, and garnish with sesame seeds if desired.
6. Serve immediately.

Nutritional Value:
Calories 360 | Fat 14g | Saturated Fat 2g | Cholesterol 0mg | Sodium 400mg | Carbohydrate 45g | Fiber 8g | Added Sugar 0g | Protein 12g | Calcium 60mg | Potassium 550mg | Iron 2.5mg | Vitamin D 0mcg

Split Pea Green Goddess Bowl

Prep Time: 10 minutes | **Cooking Time**: 30 minutes | **Total Time**: 40 minutes | **Serving**: 2 | **Cooking Difficulty**: Easy

Ingredients:

- 1/2 cup split peas, cooked
- 1/2 cup quinoa, rinsed and cooked
- 1/4 cup steamed broccoli
- 1/4 cup avocado slices
- 1 tablespoon olive oil
- 1 tablespoon lemon juice
- 1 tablespoon tahini
- 1 clove garlic, minced
- Salt and pepper, to taste
- Fresh parsley, for garnish

Instructions:

1. Cook the split peas and quinoa according to package instructions. Set aside.
2. Steam the broccoli until tender.
3. In a small bowl, whisk together olive oil, lemon juice, tahini, garlic, salt, and pepper.
4. In a serving bowl, layer the split peas, quinoa, steamed broccoli, and avocado slices.
5. Drizzle with the tahini dressing and garnish with fresh parsley.
6. Serve immediately.

Nutritional Value:
Calories 380 | Fat 16g | Saturated Fat 2g | Cholesterol 0mg | Sodium 200mg | Carbohydrate 50g | Fiber 12g | Added Sugar 0g | Protein 15g | Calcium 70mg | Potassium 600mg | Iron 4mg | Vitamin D 0mcg

Navy Bean Harvest Plate

Prep Time: 10 minutes | **Cooking Time**: 30 minutes | **Total Time**: 40 minutes | **Serving**: 2 | **Cooking Difficulty**: Easy

Ingredients:

- 1/2 cup cooked navy beans
- 1/2 cup roasted sweet potatoes
- 1/4 cup roasted Brussels sprouts
- 1/4 cup sautéed kale
- 1 tablespoon olive oil
- 1 teaspoon balsamic vinegar
- Salt and pepper, to taste
- Fresh thyme, for garnish

Instructions:

1. Roast the sweet potatoes and Brussels sprouts at 400°F (200°C) for 20-25 minutes until golden.
2. Sauté the kale in olive oil over medium heat until wilted.
3. In a serving plate, arrange the navy beans, roasted sweet potatoes, roasted Brussels sprouts, and sautéed kale.
4. Drizzle with balsamic vinegar, season with salt and pepper, and garnish with fresh thyme.
5. Serve warm.

Nutritional Value:

Calories 350 | Fat 12g | Saturated Fat 1.5g | Cholesterol 0mg | Sodium 220mg | Carbohydrate 55g | Fiber 14g | Added Sugar 0g | Protein 12g | Calcium 80mg | Potassium 700mg | Iron 4mg | Vitamin D 0mcg

Mung Bean Asian Fusion Bowl

Prep Time: 10 minutes | **Cooking Time**: 20 minutes | **Total Time**: 30 minutes | **Serving**: 2 | **Cooking Difficulty**: Easy

Ingredients:

- 1/2 cup cooked mung beans
- 1/2 cup cooked jasmine rice
- 1/4 cup shredded carrots
- 1/4 cup sautéed mushrooms
- 1 tablespoon soy sauce (low sodium)
- 1 tablespoon sesame oil
- 1 teaspoon rice vinegar
- 1 teaspoon sesame seeds (optional, for garnish)

Instructions:

1. Cook the mung beans and jasmine rice according to package instructions. Set aside.
2. Sauté the mushrooms in sesame oil over medium heat until browned.
3. In a serving bowl, layer the mung beans, jasmine rice, shredded carrots, and sautéed mushrooms.
4. Drizzle with soy sauce and rice vinegar, then toss lightly.
5. Garnish with sesame seeds and serve immediately.

Nutritional Value:

Calories 320 | Fat 10g | Saturated Fat 1.5g | Cholesterol 0mg | Sodium 350mg | Carbohydrate 45g | Fiber 7g | Added Sugar 0g | Protein 10g | Calcium 50mg | Potassium 450mg | Iron 3mg | Vitamin D 0mcg

Lima Bean Garden Plate

Prep Time: 10 minutes | **Cooking Time:** 25 minutes | **Total Time:** 35 minutes | **Serving:** 2 | **Cooking Difficulty:** Easy

Ingredients:

- 1/2 cup cooked lima beans
- 1/4 cup roasted zucchini
- 1/4 cup roasted bell peppers
- 1/4 cup fresh spinach
- 1 tablespoon olive oil
- 1 tablespoon lemon juice
- 1 teaspoon oregano
- Salt and pepper, to taste
- Fresh parsley, for garnish

Instructions:

1. Roast the zucchini and bell peppers at 400°F (200°C) for 20 minutes until tender.
2. In a serving plate, arrange the cooked lima beans, roasted zucchini, roasted bell peppers, and fresh spinach.
3. Drizzle with olive oil and lemon juice, and season with oregano, salt, and pepper.
4. Garnish with fresh parsley and serve immediately.

Nutritional Value:

Calories 300 | Fat 12g | Saturated Fat 1.5g | Cholesterol 0mg | Sodium 200mg | Carbohydrate 45g | Fiber 10g | Added Sugar 0g | Protein 12g | Calcium 70mg | Potassium 650mg | Iron 3.5mg | Vitamin D 0mcg

Mixed Legume Protein Bowl

Prep Time: 10 minutes | **Cooking Time:** 15 minutes | **Total Time:** 25 minutes | **Serving:** 2 | **Cooking Difficulty:** Easy

Ingredients:

- 1/4 cup black beans, cooked
- 1/4 cup kidney beans, cooked
- 1/4 cup chickpeas, cooked
- 1/4 cup quinoa, cooked
- 1/4 cup shredded cabbage
- 1 tablespoon olive oil
- 1 tablespoon apple cider vinegar
- 1/2 teaspoon Dijon mustard
- Salt and pepper, to taste
- Fresh cilantro, for garnish

Instructions:

1. Cook the quinoa according to package instructions. Set aside.
2. In a serving bowl, layer the black beans, kidney beans, chickpeas, quinoa, and shredded cabbage.
3. In a small bowl, whisk together olive oil, apple cider vinegar, Dijon mustard, salt, and pepper.
4. Drizzle the dressing over the bowl and toss lightly.
5. Garnish with fresh cilantro and serve immediately.

Nutritional Value:

Calories 360 | Fat 12g | Saturated Fat 1.5g | Cholesterol 0mg | Sodium 250mg | Carbohydrate 50g | Fiber 12g | Added Sugar 0g | Protein 14g | Calcium 80mg | Potassium 600mg | Iron 4mg | Vitamin D 0mcg

Honest Review of My Cookbook

I hope this message finds you well! I am reaching out to you because you recently purchased my cookbook, which focuses on nourishing, easy-to-prepare meals designed to support a balanced lifestyle.

Your feedback is incredibly important to me. If you enjoyed the recipes or found the meal prep tips helpful, I would greatly appreciate it if you could take a moment to leave an honest review on Amazon. Your insights not only help me improve future editions but also assist other readers in finding the right resources for their culinary journeys.

Thank you for your support and for being a part of this journey! If you have any questions or additional feedback, please don't hesitate to reach out.

Warm regards,

Deborah Donoho

Meal Prep Plan

Day	Breakfast	Lunch	Dinner	Snack
1	Quinoa Breakfast Bowl with Greek Yogurt and Almonds (14)	Lentil and Turkey Meatballs (20)	Chickpea and Chicken Curry (21)	Black Bean Brownie Bites (74)
2	Black Bean and Egg White Burrito (14)	Quinoa Black Bean Burgers (20)	Split Pea and Ham Soup (21)	Edamame Hummus (75)
3	Chickpea Flour Pancakes (15)	Three-Bean Turkey Chili (22)	Grilled Salmon with Lentil Salad (22)	Chickpea Energy Balls (74)
4	Lentil and Spinach Breakfast Patties (15)	Turkey and White Bean Stew (23)	Tempeh Taco Bowl (23)	Lentil Crackers (75)
5	Chia Seed Protein Pudding (16)	Black Bean and Sweet Potato Enchiladas (24)	Tofu and Edamame Stir-Fry (25)	Three Bean Dip (76)
6	Steel Cut Oats with Hemp Seeds and Berries (16)	Baked Cod with Black-Eyed Peas (25)	Chicken and Chickpea Tagine (26)	Roasted Lupini Beans (76)
7	Tempeh Breakfast Scramble (17)	Seitan and Navy Bean Stew (26)	Tuna and Cannellini Bean Salad (27)	Spiced Roasted Chickpeas (78)

8	Black Bean Breakfast Bowl (17)	Bison and Kidney Bean Chili (27)	Shrimp and Edamame Quinoa Bowl (28)	Quinoa Protein Bars (77)
9	Protein-Packed Overnight Oats (18)	Moroccan Lentil Meatballs (28)	Turkey and Black Bean Stuffed Peppers (29)	Black-Eyed Pea Fritters (77)
10	Edamame Toast with Poached Eggs (18)	Tofu and Mung Bean Curry (29)	Lamb and Lima Bean Stew (30)	Tempeh "Wings" (76)
11	Quinoa Breakfast Bowl with Greek Yogurt and Almonds (14)	Red Lentil and Cauliflower Dal (32)	Chickpea and Spinach Curry (32)	Black Bean Brownie Bites (74)
12	Black Bean and Egg White Burrito (14)	Three Bean Veggie Burgers (33)	Tempeh and Black Bean Tacos (33)	Edamame Hummus (75)
13	Chickpea Flour Pancakes (15)	Quinoa-Stuffed Eggplant (34)	Bean and Barley Buddha Bowl (34)	Chickpea Energy Balls (74)
14	Lentil and Spinach Breakfast Patties (15)	Lentil Shepherd's Pie (35)	Tofu and Edamame Noodle Bowl (35)	Lentil Crackers (75)
15	Chia Seed Protein Pudding (16)	Black Bean and Sweet Potato Patties (36)	Split Pea and Mushroom Loaf (37)	Three Bean Dip (76)
16	Steel Cut Oats with Hemp Seeds and Berries (16)	Grilled Chicken and Lentil Salad (38)	Three Bean Power Bowl (38)	Roasted Lupini Beans (76)

17	Tempeh Breakfast Scramble (17)	Quinoa Chickpea Tabbouleh (39)	Tuna and White Bean Niçoise (39)	Quinoa Protein Bars (77)
18	Black Bean Breakfast Bowl (17)	Tempeh and Black Bean Taco Salad (40)	Edamame and Salmon Poke Bowl (40)	Black-Eyed Pea Fritters (77)
19	Protein-Packed Overnight Oats (18)	Chicken and Navy Bean Greek Salad (41)	Lentil and Grilled Halloumi Bowl (41)	Spiced Roasted Chickpeas (78)
20	Edamame Toast with Poached Eggs (18)	Turkey and Garbanzo Mediterranean Salad (42)	Tofu and Mung Bean Asian Slaw (42)	Black Bean Brownie Bites (74)
21	Quinoa Breakfast Bowl with Greek Yogurt and Almonds (14)	Moroccan Chickpea Soup (44)	Black Bean and Turkey Chowder (44)	Chickpea Energy Balls (74)
22	Black Bean and Egg White Burrito (14)	Red Lentil and Quinoa Soup (45)	Navy Bean and Chicken Stew (45)	Lentil Crackers (75)
23	Chickpea Flour Pancakes (15)	Split Pea and Ham Hock Soup (46)	Three Bean Vegetable Soup (46)	Quinoa Protein Bars (77)
24	Lentil and Spinach Breakfast Patties (15)	Lentil and Barley Minestrone (47)	White Bean and Turkey Sausage Soup (47)	Spiced Roasted Chickpeas (78)
25	Chia Seed Protein Pudding (16)	Kidney Bean and Beef Chili (48)	Mung Bean and Tofu Hot Pot (48)	Black-Eyed Pea Fritters (77)

26	Steel Cut Oats with Hemp Seeds and Berries (16)	Turkey and Black Bean Enchilada Casserole (50)	Lentil and Sweet Potato Shepherd's Pie (50)	Chickpea Energy Balls (74)
27	Tempeh Breakfast Scramble (17)	Chickpea and Chicken Bake (51)	Quinoa Black Bean Mexican Casserole (51)	Black Bean Brownie Bites (74)
28	Black Bean Breakfast Bowl (17)	Tuna and White Bean Pasta Bake (52)	Three Bean and Turkey Tamale Pie (52)	Lentil Crackers (75)
29	Protein-Packed Overnight Oats (18)	Tempeh and Navy Bean Gratin (53)	Edamame Rice Casserole (54)	Spiced Roasted Chickpeas (78)
30	Edamame Toast with Poached Eggs (18)	Lima Bean and Ham Layer Bake (54)	Red Lentil Moussaka (55)	Quinoa Protein Bars (77)
31	Quinoa Breakfast Bowl with Greek Yogurt and Almonds (14)	Farro Black Bean Power Bowl (56)	Barley Chickpea Buddha Bowl (56)	Black Bean Brownie Bites (74)
32	Black Bean and Egg White Burrito (14)	Quinoa Edamame Protein Bowl (57)	Brown Rice Lentil Energy Bowl (57)	Chickpea Energy Balls (74)
33	Chickpea Flour Pancakes (15)	Bulgur White Bean Mediterranean Bowl (58)	Millet Black-Eyed Pea Soul Bowl (58)	Lentil Crackers (75)
34	Lentil and Spinach Breakfast Patties (15)	Wild Rice Tempeh Harvest Bowl (59)	Spelt Bean Burrito Bowl (59)	Spiced Roasted Chickpeas (78)

35	Chia Seed Protein Pudding (16)	Amaranth Chickpea Breakfast Bowl (60)	Teff Lentil Ancient Grain Bowl (60)	Black Bean Brownie Bites (74)
36	Steel Cut Oats with Hemp Seeds and Berries (16)	Tempeh Black Bean Collard Wrap (62)	Chickpea "Tuna" Salad Sandwich (62)	Chickpea Energy Balls (74)
37	Tempeh Breakfast Scramble (17)	Lentil Walnut Burger (63)	Turkey Bean Sprout Wrap (63)	Lentil Crackers (75)
38	Black Bean Breakfast Bowl (17)	White Bean and Tuna Pita (64)	Edamame Hummus Veggie Wrap (64)	Quinoa Protein Bars (77)
39	Protein-Packed Overnight Oats (18)	Black Bean and Quinoa Burrito (65)	Navy Bean Chicken Salad Sandwich (65)	Spiced Roasted Chickpeas (78)
40	Edamame Toast with Poached Eggs (18)	Red Lentil Falafel Wrap (66)	Split Pea Patty Sandwich (66)	Black-Eyed Pea Fritters (77)
41	Quinoa Breakfast Bowl with Greek Yogurt and Almonds (14)	Lentil Bolognese (68)	Chickpea Pasta with White Beans (68)	Chickpea Energy Balls (74)
42	Black Bean and Egg White Burrito (14)	Black Bean Pasta Primavera (69)	Edamame Noodle Stir-Fry (69)	Black Bean Brownie Bites (74)
43	Chickpea Flour Pancakes (15)	Red Lentil Penne with Turkey (70)	Three Bean Pasta Salad (70)	Lentil Crackers (75)

44	Lentil and Spinach Breakfast Patties (15)	Tempeh Marinara with Legume Pasta (71)	Navy Bean Mac and Cheese (71)	Quinoa Protein Bars (77)
45	Chia Seed Protein Pudding (16)	Mung Bean Glass Noodle Bowl (72)	Lima Bean Pasta Alfredo (72)	Spiced Roasted Chickpeas (78)
46	Steel Cut Oats with Hemp Seeds and Berries (16)	Black Bean Brownie Bites (74)	Chickpea Energy Balls (74)	Edamame Hummus (75)
47	Tempeh Breakfast Scramble (17)	Lentil Crackers (75)	Quinoa Protein Bars (77)	Three Bean Dip (76)
48	Black Bean Breakfast Bowl (17)	Edamame Hummus (75)	Black Bean Brownie Bites (74)	Quinoa Protein Bars (77)
49	Protein-Packed Overnight Oats (18)	Black Bean Brownie Bites (74)	Lentil Crackers (75)	Edamame Hummus (75)
50	Edamame Toast with Poached Eggs (18)	Chickpea Energy Balls (74)	Lentil Crackers (75)	Three Bean Dip (76)
51	Quinoa Breakfast Bowl with Greek Yogurt and Almonds (14)	Lentil Crackers (75)	Black Bean Brownie Bites (74)	Edamame Hummus (75)
52	Black Bean and Egg White Burrito (14)	Quinoa Protein Bars (77)	Three Bean Dip (76)	Black-Eyed Pea Fritters (77)

53	Chickpea Flour Pancakes (15)	Lentil and Turkey Meatballs (20)	Chickpea and Chicken Curry (21)	Edamame Hummus (75)
54	Lentil and Spinach Breakfast Patties (15)	Quinoa Black Bean Burgers (20)	Split Pea and Ham Soup (21)	Black Bean Brownie Bites (74)
55	Chia Seed Protein Pudding (16)	Three-Bean Turkey Chili (22)	Grilled Salmon with Lentil Salad (22)	Chickpea Energy Balls (74)
56	Steel Cut Oats with Hemp Seeds and Berries (16)	Turkey and White Bean Stew (23)	Tempeh Taco Bowl (23)	Lentil Crackers (75)
57	Tempeh Breakfast Scramble (17)	Black Bean and Sweet Potato Enchiladas (24)	Tofu and Edamame Stir-Fry (25)	Spiced Roasted Chickpeas (78)
58	Black Bean Breakfast Bowl (17)	Baked Cod with Black-Eyed Peas (25)	Chicken and Chickpea Tagine (26)	Quinoa Protein Bars (77)
59	Protein-Packed Overnight Oats (18)	Seitan and Navy Bean Stew (26)	Tuna and Cannellini Bean Salad (27)	Black-Eyed Pea Fritters (77)
60	Edamame Toast with Poached Eggs (18)	Bison and Kidney Bean Chili (27)	Shrimp and Edamame Quinoa Bowl (28)	Quinoa Protein Bars (77)

Conclusion

Maintaining a high-protein, high-fiber lifestyle is a rewarding journey that benefits your health, energy levels, and overall well-being. Through mindful meal planning and meal prepping, you've learned how to incorporate a variety of nutrient-dense ingredients like legumes, whole grains, vegetables, and plant-based proteins into your daily routine. This cookbook provides you with not only delicious and easy-to-follow recipes but also the essential tools to continue making wholesome, balanced meals.

Sustaining Your High-Protein, High-Fiber Lifestyle

Consistency is key in sustaining this lifestyle. Focus on variety by rotating different sources of proteins and fibers in your meals to keep things fresh and exciting. Over time, meal prepping will become second nature, and you'll develop a greater understanding of what foods work best for your schedule, taste preferences, and nutritional needs.

A successful long-term approach to this lifestyle is about balance. Don't be afraid to indulge in your favorite foods occasionally and remember that your overall dietary pattern is what matters most.

Overcoming Common Meal Prep Challenges

1. **Time Management**: Meal prepping doesn't have to take hours. Start by prepping basics like grains, legumes, and roasted vegetables in large batches. Set aside just one or two days a week to dedicate a couple of hours to prepping your ingredients and meals.

2. **Ingredient Fatigue**: If you're tired of eating the same meals, switch up your herbs, spices, and sauces. Experiment with global flavors like Mediterranean, Mexican, or Asian-inspired dishes to keep your meals interesting.

3. **Storage Issues**: Running out of storage or dealing with food spoiling before you can eat it? Invest in high-quality airtight containers and label your meals with dates to ensure freshness. Freeze portions you won't eat within a few days.

Tips for Staying Motivated and Adjusting as You Progress

1. **Set Realistic Goals**: Start small by setting manageable goals for your meal prep and nutrition. Celebrate the small wins, whether it's successfully prepping for a week or trying new recipes.

2. **Adapt Your Plan**: As you progress, listen to your body and adjust your plan accordingly. If you need more variety, try new recipes from the book or incorporate different protein and fiber sources. If your schedule changes, adapt your meal prep to fit your new routine.

3. **Track Your Progress**: Keep a food journal or use an app to track how different foods make you feel and how they align with your goals. Tracking can help you identify patterns and stay on course.

Made in United States
Troutdale, OR
12/08/2024

26056833R20064